# Dental Management of Sleep Disorders

# Dental Management of Sleep Disorders

Ronald Attanasio, DDS, MSEd, MS
Dennis R. Bailey, DDS

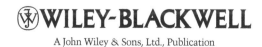

A John Wiley & Sons, Ltd., Publication

Edition first published 2010
© 2010 Blackwell Publishing

Blackwell Publishing was acquired by John Wiley & Sons in February 2007. Blackwell's publishing program has been merged with Wiley's global Scientific, Technical, and Medical business to form Wiley-Blackwell.

*Editorial Office*
2121 State Avenue, Ames, Iowa 50014-8300, USA

For details of our global editorial offices, for customer services, and for information about how to apply for permission to reuse the copyright material in this book, please see our website at www.wiley.com/wiley-blackwell.

Authorization to photocopy items for internal or personal use, or the internal or personal use of specific clients, is granted by Blackwell Publishing, provided that the base fee is paid directly to the Copyright Clearance Center, 222 Rosewood Drive, Danvers, MA 01923. For those organizations that have been granted a photocopy license by CCC, a separate system of payments has been arranged. The fee codes for users of the Transactional Reporting Service are ISBN-13: 978-0-8138-1913-6/2010.

Designations used by companies to distinguish their products are often claimed as trademarks. All brand names and product names used in this book are trade names, service marks, trademarks or registered trademarks of their respective owners. The publisher is not associated with any product or vendor mentioned in this book. This publication is designed to provide accurate and authoritative information in regard to the subject matter covered. It is sold on the understanding that the publisher is not engaged in rendering professional services. If professional advice or other expert assistance is required, the services of a competent professional should be sought.

*Library of Congress Cataloguing-in-Publication Data*

Attanasio, Ronald.
  Dental management of sleep disorders / Ronald Attanasio and Dennis R. Bailey.
     p. ; cm.
  Includes bibliographical references and index.
  ISBN-13: 978-0-8138-1913-6 (alk. paper)
  ISBN-10: 0-8138-1913-X (alk. paper)
1. Sleep disorders.   2. Dentistry.   3. Sleep apnea syndromes.   4. Bruxism.
I. Bailey, Dennis R.   II. Title.
     [DNLM: 1. Sleep Apnea Syndromes–diagnosis.   2. Sleep Apnea Syndromes–therapy.
3. Dentistry–methods.   4. Sleep Bruxism–diagnosis.   5. Sleep Bruxism–therapy.
WF 143 A883d 2010]
  RC547.A848 2010
  616.8'498–dc22

                                                                      2009026522

A catalog record for this book is available from the U.S. Library of Congress.

Set in 9.5/12 pt Palatino by Aptara® Inc., New Delhi, India

**Disclaimer**
The contents of this work are intended to further general scientific research, understanding, and discussion only and are not intended and should not be relied upon as recommending or promoting a specific method, diagnosis, or treatment by practitioners for any particular patient. The publisher and the author make no representations or warranties with respect to the accuracy or completeness of the contents of this work and specifically disclaim all warranties, including without limitation any implied warranties of fitness for a particular purpose. In view of ongoing research, equipment modifications, changes in governmental regulations, and the constant flow of information relating to the use of medicines, equipment, and devices, the reader is urged to review and evaluate the information provided in the package insert or instructions for each medicine, equipment, or device for, among other things, any changes in the instructions or indication of usage and for added warnings and precautions. Readers should consult with a specialist where appropriate. The fact that an organization or Website is referred to in this work as a citation and/or a potential source of further information does not mean that the author or the publisher endorses the information the organization or Website may provide or recommendations it may make. Further, readers should be aware that Internet Websites listed in this work may have changed or disappeared between when this work was written and when it is read. No warranty may be created or extended by any promotional statements for this work. Neither the publisher nor the author shall be liable for any damages arising herefrom. Companies and the products and instruments cited in this book are solely to assist clinicians. The authors have no financial arrangements and derive no benefits from any of these companies.

1   2010

## Dedication

If it were not for the love, understanding, and sacrifices of our respective families, the production of this book would not have been possible. This book is dedicated to them.

Ronald Attanasio is forever grateful to his wife (Elise) for faithfulness and steadfast prayers, his children (Devon, Drew and Dani, Doron, Damaris, and D'Anna) for joy and fulfillment, his novelist brother (A.A. Attanasio) for editing contributions and keeping life's perspective balanced, his deceased parents (Joseph and Louise) for having instilled the blessings of love for life and an appreciation for dedicated work ethics, and his good friends and colleagues (Dr. David Covey and Professor Caren Barnes) for their encouragement and humor.

Dennis R. Bailey is forever grateful to his wife (Donna) along with his children (Abbey, Spencer, and Mariel) who supported him in this project. As with any project of this importance, there are others who were helpful and supportive but remain unnamed. These include those who were his early mentors and teachers who influenced his desire to constantly seek more knowledge and to also share information with them in the early stages of their training. He feels blessed to have been able to contribute to the development of this text and for the opportunities that have been instrumental in his life.

# Contents

# Preface

Approximately 50–70 million people in the United States are chronic sufferers from sleep disorders, who have impaired health and daily functioning issues as a result of those disorders. The societal economic impact of sleep disorders is estimated at $16 billion annually for health care expenses and $50 billion annually regarding lost productivity. Sleep disorders are considered to be one of the most common health problems, and yet it has been demonstrated that between 82 and 98% of adults with sleep-related breathing disorders (SRBD) are undiagnosed.

As it relates to the recognition of health issues, the role of the dentist as well as auxiliary staff is becoming more apparent. No longer is the dentist solely relegated to only the management of dental structures and dental-related conditions. The dentist now has an ever-increasing role in the recognition of a patient who may be at risk for a sleep disorder. Epidemiologic data support the increasing awareness of the relationship of sleep disorders and other health issues. Clinical treatment and decision making now emphasize sound evidence based on documentation that relies on well-researched epidemiologic studies to assist in determining the coexistence of a sleep disorder, which in turn is impacting the health of a patient.

The dentist is more significant in comanaging these SRBD patients, especially those with snoring and/or obstructive sleep apnea (OSA). Not only does the dental practitioner have the opportunity to recognize a potential sleep disorder issue in their patients, but he or she also has the opportunity to interact with the sleep medicine field through both the referral and the provision of oral appliance therapy when indicated.

The present time is very exciting for dentistry regarding its contribution and participation in the field of sleep medicine. This book has been structured to provide the reader with an overview of sleep medicine as well as the assessment and management of the SRBD patient. There is an ever-increasing volume of research findings regarding sleep medicine and dentistry as each year passes. It is our intent to have readers use this book as a stepping-stone along their path of lifelong learning.

Ronald Attanasio, DDS, MSEd, MS
Dennis R. Bailey, DDS

# Section 1

## Overview of Sleep Medicine

# Impact of sleep disorders on society

## CONCEPTUAL OVERVIEW

Approximately 50–70 million people in the United States are chronic sufferers from sleep disorders, who have impaired health and daily functioning issues as a result of those disorders.[1] The societal economic impact of sleep disorders is estimated at $16 billion annually for health care expenses and $50 billion annually regarding lost productivity.[2] Sleep disorders are considered to be one of the most common health problems, and yet it has been demonstrated that between 82 and 98% of adults with sleep-related breathing disorders (SRBD) are undiagnosed.[3,4]

Sleep disorders can no longer be thought of in simple terms as having a poor night's sleep. There are currently a large number of different sleep disorders that may affect one's quality of life. In addition, there is a difference between the sleep state and the wake state. Sleep is not simply an altered state of consciousness, that is merely a difference of being asleep or being awake.

Sleep is a totally separate behavioral and physiological state that is unique and well documented, and it is defined as "a reversible behavioral state of perpetual disengagement from and unresponsiveness to the environment."[5] As such, sleep is composed of a combination of rapid eye movement (REM) and nonrapid eye movement (NREM) associated with well-defined and variable brain activity.[6] Sleep disruption and the specifically recognized sleep disorders not only may have a major impact on an individual's well-being, health status, and quality of life, but may also render significant consequences on the various areas of public health, such as accidents, mortality, morbidity, work and other daily performance, cognitive function, and utilization of health care.

# EPIDEMIOLOGY OF SLEEP DISORDERS

Epidemiology is the study of the geographic distribution and the risk factors of a particular disease,[7] and, in particular, how that disease impacts the health status of different and varying populations. Relative to sleep disorders, the origin and onset of a specific sleep disorder are often multifactorial. As such, it is essential for there to be an epidemiological awareness of both normal and abnormal sleep and wake patterns. The ultimate goal of this greater appreciation of sleep disorder epidemiology is the improvement in people's health as well as a foundation for preventative medicine and public health.

The eventual outcome of these early epidemiologic studies of normal and abnormal sleep patterns resulted in the publication of the *International Classification of Sleep Disorders* that has since been revised into its current second edition (*ICSD-2*).[8] The *ICSD-2* is the evidence-based standard for the classification, terminology, and diagnostic criteria of sleep disorders. Currently, the most common sleep disorders on the basis of epidemiologic studies are the following:[9]

1. Insomnia
2. Sleep-related breathing disorders (SRBD)
3. Restless legs syndrome (RLS)

The general onset of sleep disorders as well as their progression is, to some degree, dependent on age,[10] the presentation of being at risk for health-related consequences, and trauma. In many instances, these disorders may appear as a health issue and perhaps even some type of emotional or psychological condition. Also, the presentation of the particular health issue is sometimes not first recognized or diagnosed as maybe having an association with a sleep disorder. As an example, SRBD patients may seek treatment and utilize more health care resources for cardiovascular disease (e.g., hypertension) prior to the recognition of the SRBD as being the possible underlying cause[11] (Figure 1.1).

In addition to the overall statistics of the portion of a population that suffers from the general label of sleep disorders, the prevalence of these disorders are often referenced to the epidemiologic studies pertaining to each of the classifications recognized in the *ICSD-2*. Thus, the actual distribution of a specific sleep disorder is variable and dependent on the study that is being referenced.

Relative to the three most common sleep disorders, a 1993 study is the most frequently cited reference relative to SRBD.[3] In this study of 602 people, it was determined that 24% of men and 9% of women are at risk for SRBD, and it also demonstrated that 4% of men and 2% of women met the

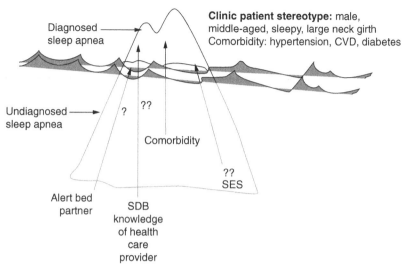

**Selection Factors**

**Figure 1.1**    Clinical recognition and diagnosis of sleep apnea. The proportion of all cases of sleep apnea is represented by the iceberg, with clinically diagnosed cases shown in the tip of the iceberg. Clinically recognized sleep apnea represents 85% of the total prevalence of sleep apnea cases that would be candidates for treatment. CVD, cerebrovascular disease; SES, socioeconomic status. "?" and "??" indicate that these particular "selection factors" are not as well known as "comorbidity" relative to the recognition and diagnosis of sleep apnea. (Young T. Rationale, design, and findings from the Wisconsin Sleep Cohort Study. Sleep Med Clin, 2009; 4(1):39. Reprinted with permission.)

criteria for SRBD, who also have daytime hypersomnolence or excessive daytime sleepiness. The correlate to this is a study that indicated 93% of females and 82% of males with moderate-to-severe SRBD are undiagnosed, and 98% of females and 90% of males who have less severe sleep apnea are undiagnosed.[4] A more recent study demonstrated that a minimum of 12–18 million people in the United States are affected by untreated SRBD.[12]

For insomnia, the prevalence may vary on the basis of the study, but, in general, it appears to be approximately 33% of the population.[13] The percentage will vary on the basis of the defined criteria that may exist as a result of the specific study parameters.

The epidemiology of RLS is estimated to be between 2.5 and 10% of the general population.[14] Many of the studies have limitations because of misdiagnoses as well as patients who may not seek medical care. With improved criteria for making a diagnosis, the recognition of RLS may actually result in an increased prevalence.

Narcolepsy is another sleep disorder that has been studied epidemiologically. At the present time, its prevalence is between 25 and 50 per 100,000 population,[15] which is a prevalence similar to multiple sclerosis.

# RISK FACTORS

There are a multitude of risk factors that may impact the onset as well as the progression of a specific sleep disorder. The risk factors may be different for each disorder, and there may also be overlapping risk factors that apply to a number of different sleep disorders. In general, the demands of modern-day life have impacted the quality of one's sleep as well as the required amounts that are deemed appropriate. In addition, the disruption of an individual's sleep can impact other family members, roommates, or one's bed partner. As an example, the results of a study pertaining to SRBD demonstrated that the snoring of one person significantly impacted the sleep of the bed partner to the point that the affected person had symptoms that were worse than those of the snorer.[16]

The risk factors frequently associated with the three most common sleep disorders are listed in Table 1.1.

# HEALTH CONSEQUENCES AND COSTS

The impact of sleep disorders on one's health can be evident in a wide range of adverse health consequences, including but not limited to hypertension,[17–19] cardiovascular diseases,[20–27] metabolic disorders such as diabetes,[28–32] gastric disorders such as gastroesophageal reflux disease,[33–36] respiratory disorders such as asthma,[37] emotional and psychological disorders,[38–41] and increased mortality rates.[42] The heightened awareness that assorted health issues potentially may arise as a result of sleep disorders is improving. Similarly, an illness or health problem may conversely impact one's sleep.

The increased risks for cardiovascular disease and elevated blood pressure associated with SRBD are well-documented. The largest and frequently cited investigation, the Sleep Heart Health Study, took place between 1995 and 1998 as a cohort study with more than 6,000 people enrolled as participants.[43] This study found that obstructive sleep apnea (OSA) along with other SRBD are risk factors for cardiovascular disease, which is inclusive of myocardial infarction and stroke. A variety of proposed mechanisms indicate that OSA and cardiovascular disease are related, and elevated blood pressure is the more common one.

Insomnia, which is the inability to fall asleep or to maintain sleep, is often associated with emotional, psychological, or depressive disorders. In addition, it can be associated with painful conditions as well as other health issues. As a sleep disorder, insomnia is the most common and may occur in conjunction with other sleep disorders such as OSA and RLS. Everyone may have insomnia at some point in their life.

Alteration in metabolic and endocrine functions is also associated with SRBD, the most prevalent of which is type 2 diabetes. It has been found

**Table 1.1**  Common risk factors for the three most common sleep disorders.

Sleep apnea and sleep-related breathing disorders
  Increase with age
  Snoring/gasping during sleep
  Associated with larger neck size
  Increase with weight
  Males greater than females
  Airway obstruction—especially tonsils, adenoids, enlarged tongue, elongated soft palate
  Hypothyroidism
  Coexisting cardiovascular disease or hypertension
  Allergy or asthma
  Family history
Insomnia
  Increases with age
  Associated with anxiety and/or depression
  Associated with pain, headaches, arthritis, temporomandibular disorder symptoms
  Dissatisfied with one's quality of sleep
  Females greater than males
  Substance abuse
  Perceives health as worse or bad
  Level of schooling
Restless legs syndrome
  Increases with age
  Worsens over time—follows a chronic course
  Males greater than females
  Use of antidepressants
  Low iron levels
  Peripheral neuropathy
  Pregnancy
  End-stage renal disease
  May coexist with sleep bruxism

that snoring alone increases the risk for type 2 diabetes independent of any other risk factors.[28]

Health issues that impact sleep are also recognized. Classically, among these are painful conditions, increased stress, and depression. These most often lead to insomnia and a decrease in sleep time and sleep quality, and, in many instances, an associated increased time in bed.

Although sleep disorders may potentially increase the risk for a multitude of health problems, it is not an absolute that a given sleep disorder will lead to any one specific health problem. The important issue is to recognize that these health problems may have an underlying sleep disorder as a contributing factor in the development or progression of a health issue. The more common health conditions associated with sleep disorders are listed in Table 1.2.

**Table 1.2** Common health issues possibly associated with a sleep disorder.

Painful conditions
Headaches
Arthritis
Fibromyalgia
Anxiety or depression
Stress
Hyperthyroidism
Pregnancy
Gastroesophageal reflux disease
Medications
Cardiovascular disease
Hypertension

There are also associations of sleep disorders with impairments in performance relative to attention and reaction time,[44–46] which could have significant impact in occupational settings. One study demonstrated that about 20% of serious injuries from motor vehicle accidents are related to driver sleepiness and not alcohol-related.[47] Other studies have indicated the equivalence of driving when sleepy as when driving under the influence of alcohol.[48,49]

A report by the National Sleep Foundation (NSF) indicated that (1) 60% of adult drivers stated that they have driven a vehicle during the past 12 months while feeling drowsy and (2) 37% self-reported that they fell asleep while driving at least 1–2 days/month.[50] The NSF report included an estimate by the National Highway Traffic Safety Administration that vehicular crashes related to driver fatigue result in a minimum estimation of $12.5 billion of monetary losses to the economy. Fiscal impact on society could be higher since there is no physical test to attribute these crashes to sleepiness.

Studies have also demonstrated the association of sleep-related fatigue and work-related injuries and fatalities.[51,52] Workers who were identified as highly fatigued had a 70% greater chance of being involved in occupation-related accidents than were workers identified with low fatigue. Another study demonstrated that workers with insomnia had a greater chance for injuries related to their occupations than workers who were identified as having good sleep.[53] Also, workers with disturbed sleep had twice as much chance of dying in a work-related accident than those who did not have sleep disturbance.[51]

Because of the increased risk for the development of health problems with sleep disorders, there may be an associated increase in health care costs as well. The presence of a sleep disorder may drive up the cost of health care in general, and it has been estimated that untreated sleep apnea may add $16 billion in medical costs annually in the United States.[2]

However, at the present time, it is unclear what the actual savings in medical costs are with the management of OSA. In a study of 31 patients diagnosed with cardiovascular disease and OSA, there was a reduction in the need for hospitalization related to the cardiovascular illness when the apnea was adequately managed.[54] An association between the severity of the sleep disorder and increased health care expenditures is possible.[55]

The costs of health care are increased by the lack of attention to the specific sleep disorder. A 1998 study demonstrated that 10 years prior to the actual diagnosis of OSA, the patients who were eventually diagnosed with OSA had incurred nearly double the costs for health care and had additional hospitalizations when compared to the matched controls.[56] As such, in many instances the sleep disorder actually precedes the onset of the specific health issue or consequence. If the sleep disorder is not discovered, then the attention to the related health issue takes precedent. This may then lead to an increase in expenditures for various testing, imaging, physician visits, hospitalization, and medication or prescription usage.

Along with the health issues that may arise, there is also an impact on one's quality of life. Studies that assessed parameters regarding quality of life demonstrated that patients with a sleep disorder feel that their quality of life is poorer than those without OSA.[57,58] When the OSA is improved with treatment, both the patient and the bed partner experience an improvement in their quality of life.[59]

## THE ROLE OF THE DENTIST

As it relates to the recognition of health issues, the role of the dentist as well as the auxiliary staff is becoming more apparent. No longer is the dentist solely relegated to only the management of dental structures and dental-related conditions. An example is the association between periodontal disease and cardiovascular disease.

Many decades ago, the dentist's role in the overall health care of the patient was initiated by performing blood pressure screenings. Patients often saw their dentist more frequently than they saw a physician, which led to the discovery of many patients who were at risk for hypertension and yet were unaware of its existence. A commentary in the *Journal of the American Dental Association* (JADA) called for an increase in the education of the dentist in biological and medical sciences.[60] This commentary directly referenced medical topics possibly related to the dentist that appeared in JADA from 2004 to 2006, including diabetes, heart disease, cardiovascular diseases, and OSA. Another commentary noted the potential for the dentist to inform patients about possible risk factors for cardiovascular disease.[61] When considering the association between SRBD and cardiovascular disease, the dentist as well as the auxiliary staff are well-poised to assist patients with their overall health.

**Table 1.3** The role of the dentist.

| Action | Indirect approach | Direct approach |
|---|---|---|
| Advise patient of potential sleep disorder | Yes | Yes |
| Obtain blood pressure and review medical history | Yes | Yes |
| Refer for further evaluation: to primary care physician or sleep specialist | Yes | Yes |
| Refer for sleep study | No | Yes |
| Based on diagnosis, actively involved with treatment | No | Yes |

The role of the dentist can potentially take on one of two roles (Table 1.3). The first, referred to as the *indirect approach*, is simply the recognition of the potential existence of a sleep disorder that may be impacting the patient's health status, and the patient is subsequently advised of the situation and referred for definitive evaluation and care. The second, referred to as the *direct approach*, is when a sleep disorder is recognized and, if appropriate, the patient is referred for more comprehensive evaluation and care. This testing often involves the primary care physician and/or sleep specialist, and the care, when deemed applicable, may also include the dentist. The dental treatment typically involves the use of an oral appliance for the management of OSA. The dentist may also be involved for treatment of a painful orofacial condition that is impacting the patient's sleep.

Regardless of the role that the dentist assumes, the initial action needs to start with the recognition of the patient who may be at risk for a health problem or who may have a health problem that may have a sleep disorder as an underlying or contributing factor.

## CONCLUSION

The dentist now has an ever-increasing role in the recognition of a patient who may be at risk for a sleep disorder. Epidemiologic data support the increasing awareness of the relationship of sleep disorders and other health issues. Clinical treatment and decision making now emphasize sound evidence based on documentation that relies on well-researched epidemiologic studies to assist in determining the coexistence of a sleep disorder, which in turn is impacting the health of a patient.

## REFERENCES

1. National Center on Sleep Disorders Research. National Sleep Disorders Research Plan. Bethesda, MD: National Heart, Lung, and Blood Institute, National Institutes of Health. 2003; vii.

2.  National Center on Sleep Disorders Research. Your Guide to Healthy Sleep. Bethesda, MD: National Heart, Lung and Blood Institute, National Center on Sleep Disorders Research, National Institutes of Health. 2005; 2.

3.  Young T, Palta M, Dempsey J, et al. The occurrence of sleep-disordered breathing among middle-aged adults. New Eng J Med. 1993; 328(17):1230–1235.

4.  Young T, Evand L, Finn L, et al. Estimation of the clinically diagnosed proportion of sleep apnea syndrome in middle-aged men and women. Sleep. 1997; 20(9):705–706.

5.  Kryger MH, Roth T, and Dement WC. Normal human sleep: an overview. In: Kryger MH, Roth T, and Dement WC, eds. Principles and Practice of Sleep Medicine. 4th ed. Philadelphia: Elsevier/Saunders. 2005; 13.

6.  Lee-Chiong TL. Sleep: A Comprehensive Handbook. 1st ed. Hoboken, New Jersey: Wiley-Liss/John Wiley & Sons. 2006; 19.

7.  Bixler EO. Preface. In: Bixler EO, guest editor. Epidemiology of Sleep Disorders: Clinical Implications, An Issue of Sleep Medicine Clinics. Vol 4. Issue 1. Philadelphia: Elsevier/Saunders. 2009; xiii.

8.  American Academy of Sleep Medicine. International Classification of Sleep Disorders, Second Edition. Westchester, IL: American Academy of Sleep Medicine. 2005.

9.  Kryger MH, Roth T, and Dement WC. Epidemiology of sleep disorders. In: Kryger MH, Roth T, and Dement WC, eds. Principles and Practice of Sleep Medicine. Philadelphia: Elsevier/Saunders. 2005; 626.

10.  Bliwise D, Carskadon M, Carey E, et al. Longitudinal development of sleep-related respiratory disturbance in adult humans. J Gerontol. 1984; 39(3):290–293.

11.  Smith R, Ronald J, Delaive K, et al. What are obstructive sleep apnea patients being treated for prior to this diagnosis? Chest. 2002; 121(7): 164–172.

12.  Young T. Rationale, design, and findings from the Wisconsin Sleep Cohort Study: toward understanding the total societal burden of sleep-disordered breathing. In: Bixler EO, guest editor. Epidemiology of Sleep Disorders: Clinical Implications, An Issue of Sleep Medicine Clinics. Vol 4. Issue 1. Philadelphia: Elsevier/Saunders. 2009; 37–46.

13.  Lee-Chiong TL. Sleep: A Comprehensive Handbook. Hoboken, New Jersey: Wiley-Liss/John Wiley and Sons. 2006; 74.

14.  Garcia-Borreguero D, Egatz R, Winkelmann J, et al. Epidemiology of restless legs syndrome: the current status. Sleep Med Rev. 2006; 10(2):153–167.

15.  Longstreth WT, Koepsell TD, Ton TG, et al. The epidemiology of narcolepsy. Sleep. 2007; 30(1):13–26.

16.  Beninati W, Harris C, Herold, D, et al. The effect of snoring and obstructive sleep apnea on sleep quality of bed partners. Mayo Clin Proc. 1999; 74:955–958.

17.  Carlson JT, Hedner JA, Ejnell H, et al. High relevance of hypertension in sleep apnea patients independent of obesity. Am J Respir Crit Care Med. 1994; 150:72–77.

18. Morrell MJ, Finn L, Kim H, et al. Sleep fragmentation, awake blood pressure, and sleep-disordered breathing in a population-based study. Am J Respir Crit Care Med. 2000; 162:2091–2096.

19. Sjöström C, Lindberg E, Elmasry A, et al. Prevalence of sleep apnoea and snoring in hypertensive men: a population based study. Thorax. 2002; 57:602–607.

20. Gami AS, Pressman G, Caples SM, et al. Association of atrial fibrillation and obstructive sleep apnea. Circulation. 2004; 110(4):364–367.

21. Dragler LF, Bortolotto LA, Lorenzi MC, et al. Early signs of atherosclerosis in obstructive sleep apnea. Am J Respir Crit Care Med. 2005; 172: 613–618.

22. Mary SM, Hung-Fat T, Lam B, et al. Endothelial function in obstructive sleep apnea and response to treatment. Am J Respir Crit Care Med. 2004; 169:348–353.

23. Lee SA, Amis TC, Byth K, et al. Heavy snoring as a cause of carotid artery atherosclerosis. Sleep. 2008; 31(9):1207–1213.

24. Eskafi M, Cline C, Nilner M, et al. Treatment of sleep apnea in congestive heart failure with a dental device. Sleep Breath. 2006; 10:90–97.

25. Mohsenin V. Is sleep apnea a risk factor for stroke? A critical analysis. Minerva Med. 2004; 95(4):291–305.

26. Culebras A. Cerebrovascular disease and the pathophysiology of obstructive sleep apnea. Curr Neurol Neurosci. Rep. 2007; 7(2):173–179.

27. Tan KCB, Chow W, Lam JCM, et al. HDL dysfunction in obstructive sleep apnea. Atherosclerosis. 2005; 184(2):377–382.

28. Al-Delaimy WK, Manson JE, Willett WC, et al. Snoring as a risk factor for type II diabetes mellitus: a prospective study. Am J Epidemiol. 2002; 155(5):387–393.

29. Lamond N, Tiggemann M, and Dawson, D. Factors predicting sleep disruption in type II diabetes. Sleep. 2000; 23(3):1–2.

30. Ayas NT. The adverse health effects of sleep restriction. Sleep Rev. 2003; (May/June):16–20.

31. Resnick HE, Redline S, Shahar E, et al. Diabetes and sleep disturbances: findings from the Sleep Heart Health Study. Diabetes Care. 2003; 26(3):702–709.

32. Punjabi NM, Sorkin JD, Katzel LI, et al. Sleep-disordered breathing and insulin resistance in middle-aged and overweight men. Am J Resp Crit Care Med. 2002; 165(5):677–682.

33. Zanation AM and Senior BA. The relationship between extraesophageal reflux (EER) and obstructive sleep apnea (OSA). Sleep Med Rev. 2005; 9:453–458.

34. Demeter P and Pap A. The relationship between gastroesophageal reflux disease and obstructive sleep apnea. J Gastroenterol. 2004; 39(9): 815–820.

35. Guda N, Parington S, Shaw MJ, et al. Unrecognized GERD symptoms are associated with excessive daytime sleepiness in patients undergoing sleep studies. Dig Dis Sci. 2007; 52(10):2873–2876.

36. Bruley des Varnes S, Errieau G, and Tessier C. Two thirds of patients with gastroesophageal reflux have nocturnal symptoms: survey by 562 general practitioners of 36663 patients. Presse Med. 2007; 36(4 Pt 1):591–597.

37. Orr WC. Gastrointestinal functioning during sleep: a new horizon in sleep medicine. Sleep Med Rev. 2001; 5(2):91–101.

38. Sharafkhaneh A, Giray N, Richardson P, et al. Association of psychiatric disorders and sleep apnea in a large cohort. Sleep. 2005; 28:1405–1411.

39. Jennum PJ and Sjol A. Cognitive symptoms in persons with snoring and sleep apnea. An epidemiologic study of 1504 women and men aged 30–60 years: the Dan-MONICA II Study. Ugeskr Laeger. 1995; 157(45):6252–6256.

40. Deldin PJ, Phillips LK, and Thomas RJ. A preliminary study of sleep-disordered breathing in major depressive disorder. Sleep Med. 2006; 7:131–139.

41. Yue W, Hao W, Lieu P, et al. A case-control study on psychological symptoms in sleep apnea–hypopnea syndrome. Can J Psychiatry. 2003; 48:318–323.

42. Partinen M, Jamieson A, Guilleminault C. Long-term outcome for obstructive sleep apnea syndrome patients: mortality. Chest. 1990; 94:1200–1204.

43. Shahar E, Whitney C, Redline S, et al. Sleep-disordered breathing and cardiovascular disease cross-sectional results of the sleep heart health study. Am J Resp Crit Care Med. 2001; 163:19–25.

44. Durmer JS and Dinges DF. Neurocognitive consequences of sleep deprivation. Sem Neurol. 2005; 25(1):117–129.

45. Van Dongen HP, Maislin G, Mullington JM, et al. The cumulative cost of additional wakefulness: dose-response effects of neurobehavioral functions and sleep physiology from chronic sleep restriction and total sleep deprivation. Sleep. 2003; 26(2):117–126.

46. Belenky G, Wesensten NJ, Thorne DR, et al. Patterns of performance degradation and restoration during sleep restriction and subsequent recovery: a sleep dose-response study. J Sleep Res. 2003; 12(1):1–12.

47. Connor J, Norton R, Ameratunga S, et al. Driver sleepiness and risk of serious injury to car occupants: population-based case control study. Brit Med J. 2002; 324(7346):1125.

48. Powell NB, Schechtman KB, Riley RW, et al. The road to danger: the comparative risks of driving while sleepy. Laryngoscope. 2001; 111(5):887–893.

49. Hack MA, Choi SJ, Vijayapalan P, et al. Comparison of the effects of sleep deprivation, alcohol and obstructive sleep apnoea (OSA) on simulated steering performance. Respir Med. 2001; 95(7):594–601.

50. National Sleep Foundation. National Sleep Foundation 2007 State of States Report on Drowsy Driving. 2007; 3.

51. Akerstedt T, Fredlund P, Gillberg M, et al. A prospective study of fatal occupational accidents—relationship to sleeping difficulties and occupational factors. J Sleep Res. 2002; 11(1):68–71.

52. Swaen GMH, Van Amelsvoort LGPM, Bultmann U, et al. Fatigue as a risk factor for being injured in an occupational accident: results from the Maastricht Cohort Study. Occup Environ Med. 2003; 60(Suppl 1):88–92.

53. Leger D, Guilleminault C, Bader G, et al. Medical and socio-professional impact of insomnia. Sleep. 2002; 25(6):625–629.

54. Peker Y, Hedner J, and Bende M. Reduced hospitalization with cardiovascular and pulmonary disease in obstructive sleep apnea patients on nasal CPAP treatment. Sleep. 1997; 20:645–653.

55. Position Statement of the American Academy of Sleep Medicine. Cost justification for diagnosis and treatment of obstructive sleep apnea. Sleep. 2000; 23(8):1017–1018.

56. Ronald J, Delaive K, Roos L, et al. Obstructive sleep apnea patients use more health care resources ten years prior to diagnosis. Sleep Res Online. 1998; 1(1):71–74.

57. Yang EH, Hla KM, McHorney CA, et al. Sleep apnea and quality of life. Sleep. 2000; 23(4):535–541.

58. Lacasse Y, Godbout C, and Series F. Health-related quality of life in obstructive sleep apnoea. Eur Respir J. 2002; 19(3):499–503.

59. Parish JM and Lyng PJ. Quality of life in bed partners of patients with obstructive sleep apnea or hypopnea after treatment with continuous positive airway pressure. Chest. 2003; 124(3):942–947.

60. Baum BJ. Inadequate training in the biological sciences and medicine for dental students: an impending crisis for dentistry. JADA. 2007; 138(1):16–26.

61. Glick M. The health of the nation. Why you should care. JADA. 2007; 138(2):144–146.

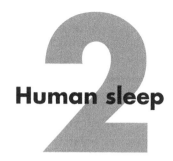

# Human sleep

## CONCEPTUAL OVERVIEW

Sleep is a universal necessity of humans, and approximately one-third of the human life is spent in the sleep state. Disruption and/or depravation of sleep typically results in adverse physiologic effects.

Despite large amounts of research and investigation into the true definition of sleep, the complete purpose for sleep is not fully understood. It is known, though, that adequate sleep is needed to maintain alertness, heal the body, and assist with memory and learning. Also, the physiologic and neurochemical activities needed for the sleep and awake states are better understood. However, the complexity and study of sleep require a comprehensive understanding of the physiology, neuroanatomy, neurochemistry, and associated mechanisms by which these areas interact.

## NORMAL SLEEP

Normal sleep can be viewed from two aspects: (1) the actual distribution of sleep cycles relative to nonrapid eye movement (NREM) and rapid eye movement (REM), and (2) the neurotransmitters that affect regulation of the sleep–wake cycle. Each of these areas changes as the human progresses from infancy to elderly.

### NREM and REM sleep

Structural characteristics of normal sleep can be referred to as sleep architecture, which comprises two distinct states: NREM, which is subdivided into Stages 1–4; and REM.[1,2] NREM and REM sleep occur in varying proportions during a sleep period, and they also alternate in a cyclical fashion with each other throughout sleep. In addition, their proportional distribution during sleep changes with age.

The typical pattern in normal sleep is for the individual to progress from wakefulness to the NREM sleep state, followed by the REM sleep state, and then cyclically alternating between REM and NREM stages. Overall, a night of sleep comprises about 75–80% of NREM sleep and 20–25% of REM sleep. When this cycling becomes irregular and/or there is a deprivation of NREM sleep stages, such as what occurs with narcolepsy, sleep disorders can develop.

Muscle activity during sleep also varies depending on REM or NREM sleep. In REM sleep, there appears to be an increase in activity in the motor centers of the brain, but there is active inhibition that is exerted on these motor neurons.

In NREM sleep, muscle activity is decreased with the maximum effect during the more restorative Stages 3 and 4.

## NREM sleep

NREM sleep has historically been subdivided into four distinct stages on the basis of characteristic brain wave and physiologic activities ever since it was initially observed and measured through electroencephalography (EEG): NREM Stage 1, NREM Stage 2, NREM Stage 3, and NREM Stage 4 (Figure 2.1).[3,4]

These four stages of NREM sleep are typically defined as follows:

Stage 1: This stage reflects a change in brain wave activity from rhythmic alpha waves to mixed-frequency waves as the individual passes from wakefulness to the initiation of sleep. NREM Stage 1 comprises about 2–5% of the total sleep time, and it is considered to be a drowsy or light sleep stage from which one can usually be awakened easily. Sudden muscle contractions can occur in this stage, and the individual may also experience a sensation of falling.

Stage 2: Although this begins to be a deeper stage of sleep with a reduction of heart rate and body temperature, it is still regarded to be light with mixed-frequency EEG activity. He or she can again be easily aroused or awakened, although an additional amount of stimulus is needed as compared to NREM Stage 1. This stage comprises about 45–55% of the total sleep time. Unique and significant features in the EEG activity of this stage are the presence of K-complex and sleep spindles, the latter of which has been postulated to being associated with memory consolidation.[5] The K-complex may appear as a result of some type of stimulation, such as noise, or it may appear spontaneously.

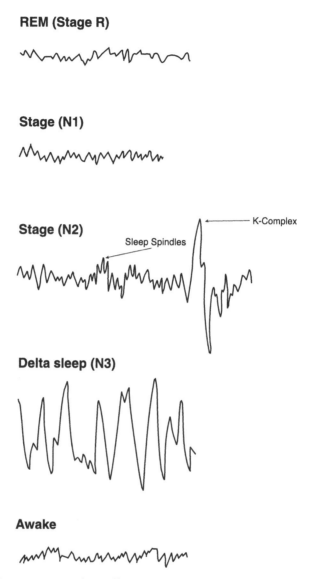

**REM (Stage R)**

**Stage (N1)**

**Stage (N2)**

Sleep Spindles

K-Complex

**Delta sleep (N3)**

**Awake**

**Figure 2.1**    EEG recordings of brain wave activity associated with their respective sleep stages.

*Stages 3 and 4:* These two NREM stages have their own unique and individually recognized brain waveforms, but they are usually viewed as one stage of sleep, being referred to as slow-wave sleep, deep sleep, or restorative sleep. Because of their unique EEG waveform, they are also known as delta sleep. Together, they comprise about 13–23% of the total sleep time. NREM Stage 4 reflects the highest threshold for awakening from sleep relative to the other NREM stages.

## REM sleep

REM sleep is also referred to as dream sleep. Although it comprises about 20–25% of the total sleep time, this state recurs several times throughout the overall cyclical activity of NREM and REM states during a sleep period. In normal sleep, each subsequent recurring REM period is longer than the prior REM period.

EEG activity is increased with a characteristic "sawtooth" waveform and can also appear similar to wakefulness relative to mixed frequency. There is a concomitant increase in heart rate, respiration, blood pressure, and jerky eye movements. During this state of increased cerebral activity, there may be an immobility or paralysis of the muscles in the limbs, which has been thought to be a preventive mechanism of the individual to not physically act out their dreams during sleep.[6] REM sleep may also be contributory to memory consolidation.[7,8]

REM sleep may be further regarded as two phases: tonic and phasic.[9] However, a typical sleep study report will not make a distinction between these two phases.

*Tonic REM* is a unique phase by virtue of the following characteristics:

- Atonia (loss of muscle tone) of the skeletal muscles that appears near paralysis;
- Desynchronized EEG activity with widespread neural activation or wake-like EEG activity.

*Phasic REM* is also unique because it occurs sporadically instead of continuously, and it reflects the following characteristics:

- Bursts of REMs in all directions;
- Transient swings in blood pressure and heart rate along with tongue movement and irregular respiration;
- Myoclonus (muscular jerks), twitching of the chin, and limb movements.

## Alternative sleep scoring/staging

In 2007, a new method of scoring sleep studies led to a revision in sleep staging,[10] and sleep study reports may increasingly refer to this nomenclature as opposed to the staging that has been historically utilized in the past (Table 2.1):

Stage W (Wakefulness)
Stage N1 (NREM1)
Stage N2 (NREM2)
Stage N3 (NREM3; this replaces NREM Stages 3 and 4)
Stage R (REM)

**Table 2.1** Comparison of sleep study scoring by stages.

| Previous scoring staging | Updated scoring staging |
| --- | --- |
| Awake | Awake |
| REM sleep | Stage R |
| NREM Stage 1 | Stage N1 |
| NREM Stage 2 | Stage N2 |
| NREM Stage 3 | Stage N3 |
| NREM Stage 4 | Stage N3 |

*Source:* Adapted from Iber C, Ancoli-Israel S, Chesson AL, et al. The AASM Manual for the Scoring of Sleep and Associated Events. Westchester, IL: American Academy of Sleep Medicine. 2007.

## Cycles and hours of sleep

Sleep patterns and architecture change for individuals throughout life. From infancy to elderly, these changes are dynamic and distinct, relative to sleep initiation, sleep maintenance, and the amount of time for each sleep stage.[11,12]

During normal sleep, the human typically cycles through the NREM and REM sleep stages four to six times per sleep period. In the adult, regardless of the age, these stages occur at about 90-minute intervals. In children, these stages are shorter and occur at about 50- to 60-minute intervals. In addition, children have different proportions of REM and NREM sleep as well as different numbers of hours of sleep. A newborn typically sleeps 16–18 hours, and 50% of this sleep time is REM sleep. Slow-wave sleep (NREM Stages 3 and 4) is at its maximum in young children since this is when growth hormone is secreted.

As we age, slow-wave sleep decreases, which appears to begin after adolescence. After the age of 70, slow-wave sleep is minimal or, in some cases, nonexistent. In addition, the elderly spend more time in bed and less time actively sleeping (Figures 2.2 and 2.3).

As people become elderly, they often begin to adjust the time that they go to bed to an earlier and earlier hour.[13] The result is that they have the increased potential to wake up earlier in the morning, which is a condition termed advanced sleep phase syndrome.[14] In this syndrome, the individual is purposely adjusting the sleep–wake schedule by attempting to initiate sleep in advance of the circadian rhythm. As such, the intentional adjustment is not synchronized with this internal biological rhythm.[15]

With the aging process, the typical sleep architecture becomes more fragmented with increased awakenings or arousals during the sleep period[16] and people tend to subsequently have an increased risk for sleep disorders,[17,18] including sleep-related breathing disorders (SRBD) and insomnia.[19] With SRBD, the musculature that supports the airway

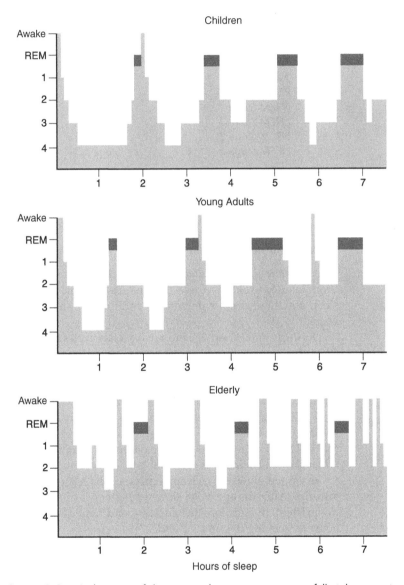

**Figure 2.2** Architecture of sleep stages by age groups over a full night at varying hours of sleep for children, young adults, and elderly. (Kales A and Kales JD. Sleep disorders: recent findings in diagnosis and treatment of disturbed sleep. New Eng J Med. 1974; 290:487. Reprinted with permission.)

becomes more relaxed during sleep, and this lends itself to increased collapsibility. Therefore, as one's age increases, the potential risk for SRBD is increased. The role of the dentist is significant for the recognition of obstructive sleep apnea (OSA) and for the management of this sleep disorder with oral appliance therapy.

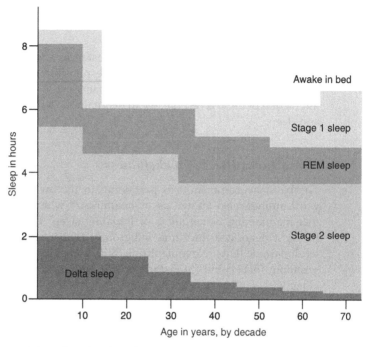

**Figure 2.3**    Sleep by decades. It shows the amount of sleep by stages over a lifetime and how these stages tend to change with age.

The number of hours of sleep that is considered to be optimal also varies with age. Infants and young children require more sleep time as compared to teenagers and adults (Table 2.2).

## Neurotransmitters of wakefulness and sleep

The role of neurotransmitters in both the sleep and awake states is a complex topic. Because of their varying levels and interaction throughout the

**Table 2.2**    Optimal hours of sleep on the basis of age.

| Age by years | Optimal hours |
| --- | --- |
| 1–3 | 12–14 |
| 3–5 | 11–13 |
| 5–12 | 10–11 |
| Teenagers | 8.5–9.5 |
| Adults | 7–9 |

*Source:* Adapted from the National Sleep Foundation. Available at www.NSF.com, 2009.

24-hour period that impacts their function, many of the neurotransmitters may appear to have contradictory functions by impacting sleep as well as wakefulness.

The interaction of these various substances (neurohormones, neuro-modulators, and neurotransmitters) is responsible for maintaining wakefulness and initiating sleep. No one substance acts alone. Rather, a complex interaction of these is responsible to maintain the two states of wakefulness and sleep.

## Neurotransmitters of wakefulness

The basic neurotransmitters pertaining to the awake state are the biogenic amines, also known as monoamines,[20] which have the role of either maintaining wakefulness or initiating sleep. These monoamines are further categorized into three subgroups: (1) catecholamines, in particular dopamine (DA), norepinephrine (NE), and epinephrine (adrenalin); (2) serotonin (5HT); and (3) histamine. The monoamines DA, NE, and 5HT along with another neurotransmitter, acetylcholine, have their origin in the brain stem, whereas histamine originates from the hypothalamus.

### Acetylcholine

This neurotransmitter is predominately for vigilance and cortical activation. It is found at the neuromuscular junctions in the sympathetic, parasympathetic, and central nervous systems. Acetylcholine is considered to have excitatory properties, and it also plays a role in the precipitation of REM sleep, especially the phasic state. In addition, it is critical for memory function.[21]

### Catecholamines

Catecholamines are found to be necessary for arousal and wakefulness, and each has unique properties:

*Dopamine* maintains wakefulness and can impact one's behavior. A reduction in dopamine is frequently associated with movement disorders.

*Norepinephrine* maintains EEG activity.

*Epinephrine* is unique because it is blood-borne and is only found to be at low levels in the brain. It is released from the adrenal medulla and is not known to cross the blood–brain barrier. Epinephrine is theorized to impact the sleep–wake cycle through autonomic and neuroendocrine regulation.

### Serotonin (5HT)

This neurotransmitter is recognized for a wide variety of functions that are associated with mood, depression, pain, headache, and sleep. It is found to be excitatory and can impact the awake state. However, its main role is to promote deep sleep.

### Histamine

The main function of histamine is to maintain quiet wakefulness. The role of histamine was not known until it was recognized that antihistamine-containing medications could produce sleepiness. Further investigation led to the discovery of the role of histamine in the promotion of wakefulness and vigilance. It functions in a fashion similar to norepinephrine by promoting cortical activation during wakefulness.

### Orexin/Hypocretin

Recently, the role of orexin (hypocretin) has also been uncovered as a neurochemical that maintains wakefulness.[22] Each of these was discovered at about the same time by two different research groups, and hence the two different names for the same neurochemical. Its role is to maintain and stabilize wakefulness as well as vigilance. More important, a reduction in the presence of orexin/hypocretin is implicated in the clinical presentation of narcolepsy. Consequently, specific medications designed to influence the release of orexin/hypocretin are used for the management of narcolepsy by maintaining wakefulness and vigilance.

### Cortisol

Cortisol is a hormone that is present to maintain wakefulness. This chemical substance is released by the adrenal glands and is oftentimes associated with stress. It also plays a role in maintaining alertness and may be increased in the early morning hours to promote wakefulness. However, because it will be increased with stress, it may also be associated with depression and insomnia.

### Glutamate

Glutamate is a fairly significant excitatory neurotransmitter in the brain that is associated with normal brain function, and it has a basic role in the activity of the waking brain. It is present mostly during wakefulness when the largest amounts can be found.[23]

## Neurotransmitters and sleep

There are a number of neurotransmitters that promote sleep, including the following.

### GABA

Gama-aminobutyric acid or $\gamma$-aminobutyric acid (GABA) is the main neurotransmitter of sleep, and it is released from the hypothalamus. With its greatest influence at the posterior hypothalamus, GABA inhibits the activating systems, hence promoting sleep.[20] Medications designed to promote sleep, such as Ambien, Sonata, and Lunesta, do so by causing the release of GABA. Benzodiazepine-type medications are also known to increase GABA, which accounts for their sedating effects. GABA is synthesized from glutamate.

### Adenosine

Adenosine is not a classic neurotransmitter. Associated with ongoing activity, it may accrue over time as a by-product of degradation from ATP. The concentration of adenosine increases with prolonged wakefulness and decreases during sleep,[24] and it is purported to be a key neurotransmitter in the homeostatic regulation of sleep. Adenosine seems to have an inhibitory affect in the central nervous system on acetylcholine and glutamate. In addition, it has the role of facilitating sleep along with GABA, which is exemplified by the fact that caffeine (methylxanthine) blocks adenosine receptors, thus explaining the role of caffeine as a stimulant.

### Serotonin

Serotonin plays a role in the control of many different functions. It is produced from tryptophan in the pineal gland of the brain, where serotonin is further affected by norepinephrine, which in turn leads to the production of melatonin.[20] The role of serotonin in sleep is, therefore, directly linked to the release of melatonin. As such, the role of serotonin is related to its impact on other neurotransmitters in either an inhibitory or stimulating fashion, which accounts for its relationship with the sleep and awake states.

About 90% of serotonin is actually produced in the intestine, and the remaining 10% is found in the brain and the platelets.[25]

## Other sleep-inducing factors

### Melatonin

Melatonin is a hormone that is released by the pineal gland in the brain and its major impact is on the circadian rhythm. As such, there is an association of light with the release of melatonin. Light that penetrates the eye terminates the release of melatonin. As darkness approaches, the stimulus to release melatonin increases, which promotes the sleep state.

The neurologic pathway related to the release of melatonin is not a direct one (Figure 2.4). The release of melatonin is initiated by the absence of light penetrating the eye, which then triggers neural activity that proceeds from the suprachiasmatic nucleus in the brain stem to the hypothalamus. The signal subsequently travels into the superior cervical nucleus of the spinal column and subsequently to the pineal gland.

### Insulin

Insulin is known to have slow-wave (NREM Stages 3 and 4) sleep-inducing properties.[26] Recently, insulin receptors have been found in the brain,

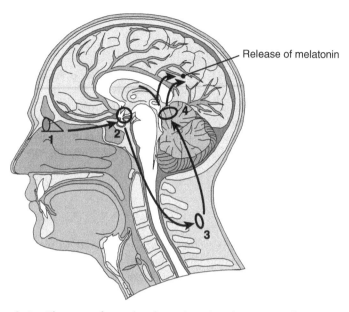

Release of melatonin

**Figure 2.4**    The route of neural pathway based on the amount of light entering the eye to get to the brain to impact the release of melatonin from the pineal gland to promote sleep.

which accounts for insulin's role in promoting sleep. One study has proposed a type of insulin dependence associated with the brain that has been termed diabetes type 3.[27] The findings are preliminary and appear to provide evidence of a relationship between sleep deprivation and Alzheimer's disease.

### Muramyl peptides

These peptides originate in the gut, and they appear to have the ability to promote sleep by stimulating the production of interleukins that are known to promote slow-wave deep sleep.[26]

## ANATOMY AND FUNCTION OF THE AIRWAY

The anatomy of the airway from the dentist's perspective is mainly focused on the upper airway, especially the musculature that directly controls airway function. These muscle groups have been categorized by anatomical location,[28] and these same muscles are employed in the function of speaking and swallowing. In addition, the dentist should be familiar with the complex action of respiration (breathing).

**Table 2.3**  Muscles designed to elevate soft palate.

| Muscle | Action |
| --- | --- |
| Levator veli palatini | Elevates the soft palate; pulls soft palate posteriorly to close the nasopharynx |
| Tensor veli palatini | Pulls soft palate laterally |
| Musculus uvulae | Elevates the uvula; pulls uvula laterally |
| Palatopharyngeus | Helps close the nasopharynx; elevates pharynx and larynx |
| Palatoglossus | Elevates tongue; narrows oropharyngeal isthmus during swallowing |

## Soft palate

Table 2.3 identifies the muscles designed to elevate and tense the soft palate. The palatopharyngeus and palatoglossus muscles are included with the soft palate because their origin is from the palatine aponeurosis, and the control of these muscles is the same as the musculus uvulae and levator veli palatini.

## Oropharynx

The posterior portion of the airway and the tongue comprise the muscles of the oropharynx. The tongue muscles are further divided into two groups: extrinsic and intrinsic (Table 2.4).

## Hyoid

The hyoid is an integral osseous structure that supports the suprahyoid and infrahyoid muscles. The position of the hyoid relative to the mandibular

**Table 2.4**  Muscles of the tongue.

| Muscle | Action |
| --- | --- |
| Extrinsic | |
| Genioglossus | Protracts tongue; depresses tongue |
| Hyoglossus | Depresses tongue |
| Styloglossus | Retracts tongue; elevates tongue |
| Palatoglossus | Elevates tongue; narrows oropharyngeal isthmus during swallowing |
| Intrinsic | |
| Superior longitudinal | Shortens tongue; curls tongue apex upward |
| Inferior longitudinal | Shortens tongue; curls tongue apex downward |
| Transverse | Narrows tongue; lengthens tongue |
| Vertical | Broadens tongue; flattens tongue |

**Table 2.5**  Infrahyoids and suprahyoids.

| Muscle | Action |
| --- | --- |
| Infrahyoids | |
| Omohyoid | Depresses hyoid |
| Sternohyoid | Depresses hyoid |
| Sternothyroid | Depresses larynx |
| Thyrohyoid | Depresses hyoid |
| Suprahyoids | |
| Stylohyoid | Elevates hyoid; retracts hyoid |
| Mylohyoid | Elevates hyoid; elevates floor of mouth |
| Digastric | Elevates hyoid; aids in depression and retraction of mandible |
| Geniohyoid | Helps move hyoid and tongue anteriorly |

plane is of importance as a reliable predictor of the risk for OSA when viewed on a cephalometric radiograph. The muscles associated with the positioning of the hyoid are divided into two groups: the infrahyoids and the suprahyoids (Table 2.5).

## Pharynx

The pharynx is the portion of the airway that runs from the base of the tongue down to the larynx and the epiglottis (Table 2.6). Because the pharynx is unsupported, it is subject to narrowing or collapse with SRBD. The pharyngeal constrictor muscles function mainly during swallowing.

## Other airway muscle considerations

Other muscles associated with mandibular function and the cervical spine play a role in positioning the mandible and head as well as maintaining the airway both in the awake and sleep states. The muscles include the masseter, temporalis, pterygoids (lateral and medial), and the anterior and posterior cervical groups.

**Table 2.6**  Muscles of the pharynx.

| Muscle | Action |
| --- | --- |
| Superior constrictor | Constricts upper portion of pharynx |
| Middle constrictor | Constricts middle portion of pharynx |
| Inferior constrictor | Constricts lower portion of pharynx |
| Palatopharyngeus | Elevates pharynx; helps close nasopharynx |
| Salpingopharyngeus | Elevates upper and later portions of pharynx |
| Stylopharyngeus | Elevates pharynx; expands sides of pharynx (dilates pharynx) |

The two main muscles of the neck that are considered as accessory to respiration are the sternocleidomastoid (SCM) and the scalene.[29] The SCM's primary purpose is to rotate, tilt, and flex the head. They also act as accessory muscles of respiration by elevating the sternum. The scalene group causes lateral flexion of the neck, and the anterior scalene specifically elevates the first rib as well as stabilizes the upper ribs with respiration.

The primary muscles of respiration during inspiration are the diaphragm and the external intercostals. During expiration, the abdominal muscles and the internal intercostals are active.

If the airway becomes compromised during inspiration, inspiratory pressures will elevate, which will result in an increased negative pressure in the airway that further compromises and possibly even collapses the airway. Many times, the muscles that are intended to support the airway as well as tongue position can no longer maintain the airway, and further collapse is inevitable. This airway collapse occurs because the musculature relaxes during sleep, thereby further complicating the compromised airway.

## NERVE SUPPLY TO THE MUSCLES OF THE AIRWAY

The muscles that are involved with respiration are supplied by either cranial nerves or nerves that originate from the cervical spine (Table 2.7). Because of this neuromuscular relationship, the evaluation of patients with SRBD needs to include an assessment of the posture, cervical spine, and, when indicated, cranial nerves.

## BASICS OF AIRWAY DYNAMICS

The Venturi effect and the Bernoulli's principle are two basic principles of airway dynamics. According to the Venturi effect, if the diameter of a tube (e.g., the airway) is decreased, then for a given volume of fluid to pass through the tube, the velocity has to increase. This concept applies to the airway relative to snoring. The Bernoulli's principle states that as fluid flows through a tube and with an increase in the flow of that substance, there is an increase in negative pressure at the periphery. The result is an increasing potential for airway collapse.

Another concept that can be associated with airway dynamics is that of the variable resistor. As the rate of flow increases, so does the resistance to that flow. However, the classic explanation that involves airway collapse related to flow is the Starling resistor concept. In this situation, a collapsible tube is positioned between two rigid structures. Relative to respiration, the collapsible tube is the airway between the nose and the trachea. When the airflow increases and the pressure outside the tube is greater than the pressure inside the tube, there is subsequent airway collapse. In the awake state,

**Table 2.7** Nerve supply to the muscles of the upper airway.

| Nerve | Muscles supplied |
|---|---|
| Trigeminal CN V | Tensor veli palatini<br>Mylohyoid<br>Anterior belly of digastric<br>Masseter<br>Medial/lateral pterygoids<br>Temporalis |
| Facial CN VII | Stylohyoid<br>Posterior belly of diagatric |
| Glossopharyngeal CN IX | Stylopharyngeus |
| Pharyngeal plexus from vagus CN X | Musculus uvulae<br>Palaptoglossus |
| Cranial part of accessory CN XI | Palatopharyngeus<br>Levator veli palatini<br>Salpingopharyngeus<br>Superior constrictor<br>Middle constrictor |
| Spinal accessory CN XI | Sternocleidomastoid (SCM)<br>Trapezius (along with C-3 and C-4 branches) |
| Pharyngeal plexus—external laryngeal of vagus & recurrent laryngeal of vagus | Inferior constrictor |
| Hypoglossal CN XII | Genioglossus<br>Hyoglossus<br>Styloglossus<br>Superior longitudinal<br>Inferior longitudinal<br>Transverse<br>Vertical |
| C-1 follows CN XII | Thyrohyoid<br>Geniohyoid |
| Ansa cervicalis<br>  Motor component of cervical plexus (C-1 to C-4) | Omohyoid<br>Sternohyoid<br><br>Sternothyroid |
| Ventral rami<br>  C-4 to C-6 | <br>Anterior scalenes |
| C-5 to C-8 | Middle scalenes |
| C-6 to C-8 | Posterior scalenes |
| Phrenic nerve from C-3 to C-5 | Diaphragm |

*Source*: Adapted from Norton NS. Netter's Head and Neck Anatomy for Dentistry. Philadelphia: Saunders/Elsevier. 2007.

the airway is not subject to these fluctuations in the pressure, and therefore the airway remains open. However, during sleep when the airway relaxes and negative pressure increases, the transmural forces that support the airway are not capable of resisting the negative pressure, and this leads to airway obstruction. Depending on the variation in pressure during respiration, the flow through the tube (i.e., airway) may be unimpeded, cause flutter, or become blocked. This correlates with normal breathing, snoring, and obstruction associated with apnea.[30]

## NORMAL RESPIRATION

Under normal circumstances, respiration is considered to be involuntary. It is primarily under the control of the diaphragm, which is innervated by the phrenic nerve that arises from the cervical nerves C3 to C5. It is primarily the muscle fibers that cause contraction of the diaphragm. During passive breathing, the diaphragm contracts and moves downward, causing an increase in the negative pressure within the lung and the alveoli. This negative pressure causes air to flow into the lungs to fill them. In addition, this action may be impacted by the intercostal muscles and the scalenes. Expiration during quiet breathing is passive, and there is no active muscle activity. The process is related to the elastic recoil of the lungs and the rib cage.

Forced inspiration and expiration are different. With forced inspiration, the scalene and the SCM muscles are active. They impact the first and second ribs as well as the sternum, and this causes elevation of the bony cage.

Forced expiration is primarily an action of the intercostal muscles that pull the thoracic cage inward and force air out of the lungs. They prevent the increased intrathoracic pressure from causing any bulging at the intercostal spaces.

## CONCLUSION

Understanding sleep and the processes related to it is important because it helps in understanding the dynamics of sleep disorders, especially SRBD. The dentist does not have to understand the complex neurologic and neurochemical relationships that exist with sleep, but it is prudent to have an understanding of the basics, the knowledge of the relevant aspects of sleep, and the ability to recognize how normal sleep may become altered. This understanding allows the dentist to have the foundational knowledge to explain certain aspects of sleep to patients who wish to have a better appreciation of their sleep and why disruption of it is occurring.

In addition, understanding sleep and sleep disorders will enable the dentist to better communicate with physicians regarding a patient who may have sleep disorders. For the sake of the patient, the dentist should have an ever-increasing awareness of medical issues relative to their patients.

Humans spend nearly a fourth to a third of their lives sleeping. It is important to understand this process as much as the other physical conditions. The time that is spent sleeping has an important role in maintaining health, improving memory, enabling humans to learn, and maintaining alertness and vigilance while awake. Without quality sleep, the awake time, mood, and ability to function may be significantly impaired.

# REFERENCES

1. Zepelin H, Siegel JM, and Tobler I. Mammalian sleep. In: Kryger MH, Roth T, and Dement WC, eds. Principles and Practice of Sleep Medicine. 4th ed. Philadelphia: Elsevier/Saunders. 2005; 91–100.
2. Carskadon MA and Rechtschaffen A. Monitoring and staging human sleep. In: Kryger MH, Roth T, and Dement WC, eds. Principles and Practice of Sleep Medicine. 4th ed. Philadelphia: Elsevier/Saunders. 2005; 1359–1377.
3. Loomis AL, Harvey EN, and Hobart GA. Cerebral states during sleep as studied by human brain potentials. J Exp Psychol. 1937; 21(2):127–144.
4. Dement W and Kleitman N. Cyclic variations in EEG during sleep and their relation to eye movements, body motility, and dreaming. Electroenceph Clin Neurophysiol: Suppl. 1957; 9(4):673–690.
5. Gais S, Molle M, Helms K, et al. Learning-dependent increases in sleep spindle density. J Neurosci. 2002; 22(15):6830–6834.
6. Bader G, Gillberg C, Johnson M, et al. Activity and sleep in children with ADHD. Sleep. 2003; 26:A136.
7. Crick F and Mirchison G. The function of dream sleep. Nature. 1983; 304(5922):111–114.
8. Smith C and Lapp L. Increases in number of REMs and REM density in humans following an intensive learning period. Sleep. 1991; 14(4): 325–330.
9. Lee-Chiong T. Sleep: A Comprehensive Handbook. Wilmington, DE: Wiley-Liss/John Wiley & Sons Inc. 2006; 3.
10. Iber C, Ancoli-Israel S, Chesson AL, et al. The AASM Manual for the Scoring of Sleep and Associated Events. Westchester, IL: American Academy of Sleep Medicine. 2007.
11. Davis KF, Parker KP, and Montgomery GL. Sleep in infants and young children: part one: normal sleep. J Pediatr Health Care. 2004; 18(2):65–71.
12. Jenni OG and Carskadon MA. Normal human sleep at different ages: infants to adolescents. In: Sleep Research Society, eds. SRS Basics of Sleep Guide. Westchester, IL: Sleep Research Society. 2005; 11–19.
13. Duffy JF, Dijk DJ, Klerman EB, et al. Later endogenous circadian temperature nadir relative to an earlier wake time in older people. Am J Phsyiol. 1998; 275(5 Pt 2):R1478–R1487.

14. Hauri PJ, Task Force Chair. International Classification of Sleep Disorders, Second Edition. Westchester, IL: American Academy of Sleep Medicine. 2005; 121.

15. Dijk DJ, Duffy JF, and Czeisler CA. Contribution of circadian physiology and sleep homeostasis to age-related changes in human sleep. Chronobiol Int. 2000; 17(3):285–311.

16. Bliwise DL. Sleep in normal aging and dementia. Sleep. 1993; 16:40–81.

17. Ancoli-Israel S. Normal human sleep at different ages: sleep in older adults. In: Sleep Research Society, eds. SRS Basics of Sleep Guide. Westchester, IL: Sleep Research Society. 2005; 21–26.

18. Bliwise DL. Normal aging. In: Kryger MH, Roth T, and Dement WC, eds. Principles and Practice of Sleep Medicine. 4th ed. Philadelphia: Elsevier/Saunders. 2005; 24–38.

19. Redline S, Kirchner HL, Quan SF, et al. The effects of age, sex, ethnicity and sleep-disordered breathing on sleep architecture. Arch Intern Med. 2004; 164:406–418.

20. Purves D, ed. Neuroscience. Sunderland, MA: Sinauer Associates. 1977.

21. Little N. Insight Wellness Staff Article: AcetylCholine, Acetylcholine Function and Chemical Imbalance. Available at www.anxiety-and-depression solutions.com/insight_answers/acetycholine.php. Accessed December 27, 2006.

22. Kryger MH, Roth T, and Dement WC. Principles and Practice of Sleep Medicine. Philadelphia: Elsevier/Saunders. 2005; 144.

23. Kryger MH, Roth T, and Dement WC. Principles and Practice of Sleep Medicine. Philadelphia: Elsevier/Saunders. 2005; 143.

24. Lee-Chiong T. Sleep Medicine. Philadelphia: Hanley & Belfus. 2002; 2.

25. Gershon MD. The Second Brain. New York: Harper Perennial. 1998.

26. Kryger MH, Roth T, and Dement WC. Principles and Practice of Sleep Medicine. Philadelphia: Elsevier/Saunders. 2005; 147.

27. Steen E, Terry BM, Rivera EJ, et al. Impaired insulin and insulin-like growth factor expression and signaling mechanisms in Alzheimer's disease—is this type 3 diabetes? J Alzheimers Dis. 2005; 7(1):63–80.

28. Norton NS. Netter's Head and Neck Anatomy for Dentistry. Philadelphia: Saunders/Elsevier. 2007.

29. Gardner E, Gray DJ, O'Rahilly R. Anatomy: A Regional Study of Human Structure. Philadelphia: WB Saunders Co. 1969; 694.

30. Lee-Chiong T. Sleep: A Comprehensive Handbook. Wilmington, DE: Wiley-Liss/John Wiley & Sons Inc. 2006; 213–214.

# Classification of sleep disorders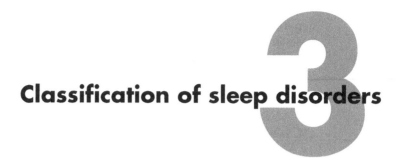

## CONCEPTUAL OVERVIEW

Although this chapter will review the overall classification of sleep disorders, the focus will primarily be on the most common adult-related types of disorders. As with any other areas or disciplines of clinical dentistry, a classification system for sleep disorders will facilitate a comprehension of the various disorders, especially with regard to signs and symptoms, pathophysiology, etiology, and clinical management.

Along with insomnia, sleep-related breathing disorders (SRBD) constitute a significant portion of sleep disorders that may be encountered in a dental clinical practice. However, for a greater appreciation of the spectrum of sleep disorders, the practitioner is encouraged to at least be familiar with the more common sleep disorders.

## CLASSIFICATION SYSTEMS

A classification system assists with the development of a differential diagnosis of any kind of health disorder.

There are four classification systems for sleep disorders that are most frequently used:

1. *Diagnostic Classification of Sleep and Arousal Disorders (DCSAD)*
2. *International Classification of Sleep Disorders, Second Edition (ICSD-2)*
3. *International Classification of Diseases (ICD)*
4. *Diagnostic and Statistical Manual of Mental Disorders (DSM)*

In general, the *DCSAD* and *ICSD-2* classification systems provide in-depth descriptive definitions that are employed for communication purposes in the clinical fields of medical sleep specialists and dentists, whereas the *ICD* versions and their numerical codes are more frequently used for medical records, billing purposes, and research focused on epidemiological studies.

## DCSAD

The *Diagnostic Classification of Sleep and Arousal Disorders (DCSAD)* was the initial classification system for sleep disorders and was first published in 1979. The *DCSAD* was subsequently used as the foundation for the formation of the other classification systems.[1]

## ICSD/ICSD-2

The American Academy of Sleep Medicine along with the Japanese Society of Sleep Research, Latin American Sleep Society, and European Sleep Research Society published the *International Classification of Sleep Disorders (ICSD): Diagnostic and Coding Manual* in 1990,[2] which was later revised in 1997. These earlier versions of the *ICSD* were utilized mostly for clinical diagnostic purposes as well as enhancement of international communication relative to research in sleep disorders. Since the pathophysiology was not well understood at that time, the *ICSD* was based on the most common symptoms of dyssomnias (insomnia and excessive daytime sleepiness (EDS)) and parasomnias (abnormal physiological events) that would take place while sleeping.

The most recent edition, *International Classification of Sleep Disorders, Second Edition (ICSD-2)*, was published in 2005.[3] This version provides a listing of the different sleep disorders as well as other diagnostic and epidemiologic information. There are 85 different sleep disorders in eight different major categories identified in the *ICSD-2* (Table 3.1).

## ICD-9-CM/ICD-10

When the World Health Organization was formed in 1948, it published the sixth edition of the *International Classification of Diseases (ICD)* for the purposes of diagnostic coding as well as collating mortality statistics regarding all medical conditions. Prior to this edition, the classification and listing of causes of death had their origins in the 1850s.[4] The *ICD* has since undergone ten revisions that include clinical modifications *(ICD-CM)*.

Sleep disorders are classified in the ninth edition, *ICD-9-CM*, as either "the specific disorders of sleep of nonorganic origin" (coding 307.4) or "the sleep disturbances" (coding 780.5).

The *ICD-10* will eventually replace the *ICD-9-CM*.

**Table 3.1** *International Classification of Sleep Disorders (ICSD-2).*

I. Insomnias
   Adjustment insomnia
   Psychological insomnia
   Paradoxical insomnia
   Idiopathic insomnia
   Insomnia due to mental disorder
   Inadequate sleep hygiene
   Insomnia due to drug or substance or alcohol use
   Insomnia due to medical condition
   Insomnia not due to substance or known physiological condition, unspecified (nonorganic insomnia)

   Physiological (organic) condition, unspecified
II. Sleep-related breathing disorders
   Primary central sleep apnea
   Cheyne–Stokes breathing pattern
   High-altitude periodic breathing
   Central apnea due to medical condition, not Cheyne–Stokes
   Central apnea due to drug or substance
   Obstructive sleep apnea, adult
   Sleep-related nonobstructive alveolar hypoventilation, idiopathic
   Sleep-related hypoventilation/hypoxemia due to pulmonary parenchymal or vascular pathology

   Sleep-related hypoventilation/hypoxemia due to lower airways obstruction
   Sleep-related hypoventilation/hypoxemia due to neuromuscular and chest wall disorders

   Other sleep-related breathing disorders
III. Hypersomnias
   Narcolepsy with cataplexy
   Narcolepsy without cataplexy
   Narcolepsy due to medical condition without cataplexy
   Narcolepsy due to medical condition with cataplexy
   Narcolepsy, unspecified
   Recurrent hypersomnia (including Kleine–Levin syndrome and menstrual-related hypersomnia)

   Idiopathic hypersomnia with long sleep time
   Idiopathic hypersomnia without long sleep time
   Behaviorally induced insufficient sleep syndrome
   Hypersomnia due to medical condition
   Hypersomnia due to drug or substance (abuse) or alcohol use
   Hypersomnia due to dug or substance (medications)
   Hypersomnia not due to substance or known physiological condition
   Physiological (organic) hypersomnia, unspecified

(Continued)

**Table 3.1**  (*Continued*)

IV.  Circadian rhythm sleep disorders
  Delayed sleep phase type
  Advanced sleep phase type
  Irregular sleep–wake rhythm
  Nonentrained type
  Jet lag type
  Shift work type
  Circadian rhythm sleep disorder due to medical condition
  Other circadian rhythm sleep disorder
  Drug or substance or alcohol use
V.  Parasomnias
  Confusional arousals
  Sleepwalking
  Sleep terrors
  REM sleep behavior disorder
  Recurrent isolated sleep paralysis
  Nightmare disorder
  Sleep-related dissociative disorders
  Sleep-related groaning
  Exploding head syndrome
  Sleep-related hallucinations
  Sleep-related eating disorder
VI.  Sleep-related movement disorders
  Restless legs syndrome
  Periodic limb movement disorder
  Sleep-related leg cramps
  Sleep-related bruxism
VII.  Isolated symptoms, apparently normal variants, and unresolved issues
  Long sleeper
  Short sleeper
  Snoring
  Sleeptalking
  Sleep starts (hypnic jerks)
  Benign sleep myoclonus of infancy
  Hypnagogic foot tremor and alternating leg muscle activation during sleep
  Propriospinal myoclonus at sleep onset
  Excessive fragmentary myoclonus
VIII.  Other sleep disorders
  Other physiological (organic) sleep disorder
  Physiological (organic) sleep disorder, unspecified
  Other sleep disorder not due to substance or physiological condition
  Environmental sleep disorder
  Other sleep disorder not due to substance or physiological condition,
  unspecified

**Table 3.1**  *(Continued)*

IX.  Sleep disorders associated with conditions classifiable elsewhere
Fatal familial insomnia
Fibromyalgia
Sleep-related epilepsy
Sleep-related headaches
Sleep-related gastroesophageal reflux disease
Sleep-related coronary artery ischemia
Sleep-related abnormal swallowing, choking, and laryngospasm
X.  Other psychiatric/behavioral disorders frequently encountered in the
differential diagnosis of sleep disorders
Mood disorders
Anxiety disorders
Selected somatoform disorders (somatization disorder, hypochondriasis)
Schizophrenia and other psychotic disorders
Selected disorders usually first diagnosed in infancy, childhood, or adolescence
(mental retardation, pervasive developmental disorders, attention deficit/
hyperactivity disorder)
Personality disorder

*Source:* International Classification of Sleep Disorders, Second Edition: Diagnostic and Coding
Manual. American Academy of Sleep Medicine. 2006.

## DSM

The American Psychiatric Association first published the *Diagnostic and Statistical Manual of Mental Disorders (DSM)* in 1952. The *DSM* has undergone several revisions since its initial publication. The *DSM Fourth Edition, Text Revision (DSM-IV-TR)* was published in 2000 and it incorporated textual descriptions for each of the sleep disorders. A 2005 publication of the classification reflects changes made to the *ICD-9-CM.*

# DEFINITIONS OF COMMON SLEEP DISORDERS (BASED ON *ICSD-2*)

Regarding frequency of sleep disorders, one report indicated that obstructive sleep apnea (OSA), narcolepsy, and restless legs syndrome (RLS) were the three most common disorders observed in a survey of sleep centers.[5] Insomnia and other sleep disorders are also considered as frequently reported or described by patients seeking care.[6]

Since sleep disorders are common in the general population, it is prudent for the dental clinician to be familiar with the definitions of these disorders. This chapter presents the definitions of common sleep disorders on the basis of the *ICSD-2* classification.

## Insomnia

Insomnia is defined by a repeated difficulty with sleep initiation, duration, consolidation, or quality that occurs despite adequate time and opportunity for sleep and results in some form of daytime impairment.[3]

The most commonly reported sleep disorder is insomnia.[6] This disorder is founded on subjective reporting by the patient, and insomnia can typically include difficulty getting to sleep, awakening from sleep earlier than the desired wake-up time, difficulty in getting back to sleep, as well as the feeling of a poor quality of sleep. These subjective complaints are reported even though the individual has had ample time for sleep, and the end result is typically EDS or fatigue along with its subsequent adverse impact on daytime function and quality of wakefulness.[7] These subjective complaints may be generally confirmed through the objective findings of a polysomnogram (PSG) sleep study,[8] but PSG is not the standard of care for the definitive diagnosis of insomnia (Table 3.2).

Although the etiology of insomnia is not completely understood, it appears to involve biological, psychological, and social elements, and it can be regarded as a condition of hyperarousal.[9]

There are 10 types of insomnia (Table 3.1), 5 of which are further described here.

**Table 3.2**  *ICSD-2 general criteria for insomnia.*

A.  A complaint of difficulty initiating sleep, difficulty maintaining sleep, or waking up too early, or sleep that is chronically nonrestorative or poor in quality. In children, the sleep difficulty is often reported by the caretaker and may consist of observed bedtime resistance or inability to sleep independently.

B.  The sleep difficulty occurs despite adequate opportunity or circumstances for sleep.

C.  At least one of the following forms of daytime impairment related to the nighttime sleep difficulty is reported by the patient:
    a.  Fatigue or malaise
    b.  Attention, concentration, or memory impairment
    c.  Social or vocational dysfunction or poor school performance
    d.  Mood disturbance or irritability
    e.  Daytime sleepiness
    f.  Motivation, energy, or initiative reduction
    g.  Proneness for errors or accidents at work or while driving
    h.  Tension headaches, or gastrointestinal symptoms in response to sleep loss
    i.  Concerns or worries about sleep.

*Source:* International Classification of Sleep Disorders, Second Edition: Diagnostic and Coding Manual. American Academy of Sleep Medicine. 2006.

**Table 3.3**  *ICSD-2* diagnostic criteria for psychophysiological insomnia.

A.  The patient's symptoms meet the criteria for insomnia.
B.  The insomnia is present for at least 1 month.
C.  The patient has evidence of conditioned sleep difficulty and/or heightened arousal in bed as indicated by one or more of the following:
   a.  Excessive focus on and heightened anxiety about sleep
   b.  Difficulty falling asleep in bed at the desired bedtime or during planned naps, but no difficulty falling asleep during other monotonous activities when not intending to fall asleep
   c.  Ability to sleep better away from home than at home
   d.  Mental arousal in bed characterized either by intrusive thoughts or a perceived inability to volitionally cease sleep-preventing mental activity
   e.  Heightened somatic tension in bed reflected by a perceived inability to relax the body sufficiently to allow the onset of sleep.
D.  The sleep disturbance is not better explained by another sleep disorder, medical or neurological disorder, mental disorder, medication use, or substance use disorder.

*Source:* International Classification of Sleep Disorders, Second Edition: Diagnostic and Coding Manual. American Academy of Sleep Medicine. 2006.

## Psychophysiological insomnia

The essential feature of psychophysiological insomnia is heightened arousal and learned sleep-preventing associations that result in a complaint of insomnia and associated decreased functioning during wakefulness.[3]

This type of insomnia involves an overconcern or worry on the individual's part relative to his or her difficulty to adequately sleep.[10,11] As such, it is a learned or behavioral insomnia since the individual is reacting to general psychologically stressful conditions that result in physical discomforts and a heightened level of arousal (Table 3.3).

## Adjustment insomnia

The essential feature of adjustment insomnia is the presence of insomnia in association with an identifiable stressor.[3]

Associated with this type of insomnia is a specific stressful situation or factor that can be psychological, physiological, environmental, or physical.[12,13] Usually, when the stressful situation resolves, so does the insomnia. Adaptation of the individual to the stress factor can also account for resolution of adjustment insomnia. As such, this type of insomnia is typically regarded as a short-term disorder, although an unaddressed stressor can cause it to develop into a more chronic condition (Table 3.4).

**Table 3.4**  *ICSD-2* diagnostic criteria for adjustment insomnia.

A.   The patient's symptoms meet the criteria for insomnia.
B.   The sleep disturbance is temporarily associated with an identifiable stressor that is psychological, psychosocial, interpersonal, environmental, or physical in nature.
C.   The sleep disturbance is expected to resolve when the acute stressor resolves or when the individual adapts to the stressor.
D.   The sleep disturbance lasts for less than 3 months.
E.   The sleep disturbance is not better explained by another sleep disorder, medical or neurological disorder, mental disorder, medication use, or substance use disorder.

*Source:* International Classification of Sleep Disorders, Second Edition: Diagnostic and Coding Manual. American Academy of Sleep Medicine. 2006.

## Inadequate sleep hygiene

The essential feature of inadequate sleep hygiene is an insomnia associated with daily living activities that are inconsistent with the maintenance of good quality sleep and full daytime alertness.[3]

Inadequate sleep hygiene is usually associated with habits or daily activities that are not conducive to sleep or good sleep quality.[14,15] Examples include (1) the intake of caffeine, alcohol, nicotine, or excess food too close to the desired initiation of sleep, (2) participating in physical exercise too close to the time of getting to sleep, and (3) a change in one's environment from travel or a change in one's work schedule, which can disrupt the body's circadian rhythms and associated sleep–wake cycle (Table 3.5).

## Insomnia due to medical condition

The essential feature of insomnia due to a medical condition is insomnia that is caused by a coexisting medical disorder or other physiologic factor.[3]

Medical conditions or neurological disorders can disrupt sleep and cause insomnia.[16,17] Examples include asthma, emphysema, bronchitis, headache, overactive thyroid, odontalgia, gastrointestinal disorders, stroke, RLS, and physical pain from fibromyalgia, myofascial pain, arthritis, temporomandibular disorders, and other medical issues.

From the dentist's perspective, the practitioner needs to discern whether a patient's chief symptoms of orofacial pain may or may not have an underlying sleep disorder as a contributing factor so that an appropriate diagnosis and management plan can be established (Table 3.6).

**Table 3.5** *ICSD-2* diagnostic criteria for inadequate sleep hygiene.

A.  The patient's symptoms meet the criteria for insomnia.
B.  The sleep disturbance is present for at least 1 month.
C.  Inadequate sleep hygiene practices are evident as indicated by the presence of at least one of the following:
    a.  Improper sleep scheduling consisting of frequent daytime napping, selecting highly variable bedtime or rising times, or spending excessive amounts of time in bed
    b.  Routine use of products containing alcohol, nicotine, or caffeine, especially in the period preceding bedtime
    c.  Engagement in mentally stimulating, physically activating, or emotionally upsetting activities too close to bedtime
    d.  Frequent use of the bed for activities other than sleep (e.g., television watching, reading, studying, snacking, thinking, planning)
    e.  Failure to maintain a comfortable sleeping environment.
D.  The sleep disturbance is not better explained by another sleep disorder, medical or neurological disorder, mental disorder, medication use, or substance use disorder.

*Source:* International Classification of Sleep Disorders, Second Edition: Diagnostic and Coding Manual. American Academy of Sleep Medicine. 2006.

## Insomnia due to a drug or substance

The essential feature of insomnia due to drug or substance abuse is a suppression or disruption of sleep caused by consumption of a prescription medication, recreational drug, caffeine, alcohol, or food item or by exposure to an environmental toxin.[3]

The ingestion or discontinuation of a drug or substance can be associated with insomnia. Examples include alcohol, caffeine, over-the-counter antihistamine cold and allergy medications, prescription medications for asthma or beta-blockers for heart conditions, as well as recreational drugs (Table 3.7).

**Table 3.6** *ICSD-2* diagnostic criteria for insomnia due to medical condition.

A.  The patient's symptoms meet the criteria for insomnia.
B.  The sleep disturbance is present for at least 1 month.
C.  The patient has a coexisting medical or physiological condition known to disrupt sleep.
D.  Insomnia is clearly associated with the medical or physiological condition. The insomnia began near the time of onset or with significant progression of the medical or physiological condition and waxes and wanes with fluctuations in the severity of this condition.
E.  The sleep disturbance is not better explained by another sleep disorder, medical or neurological disorder, or mental disorder.

*Source:* International Classification of Sleep Disorders, Second Edition: Diagnostic and Coding Manual. American Academy of Sleep Medicine. 2006.

**Table 3.7** *ICSD-2* diagnostic criteria for insomnia due to drug or substance.

A.  The patient's symptoms meet the criteria for insomnia.
B.  The sleep disturbance is present for at least 1 month.
C.  One of the following applies:
    a.  There is current ongoing dependence on or abuse of a drug or substance known to have sleep-disruptive properties either during periods of use or intoxication or during periods of withdrawal
    b.  There is current ongoing use of or exposure to a medication, food, or toxin known to have sleep-disruptive properties in susceptible individuals.
D.  The insomnia is temporarily associated with the substance exposure, use or abuse, or acute withdrawal.
E.  The sleep disturbance is not better explained by another sleep disorder, medical or neurological disorder, or mental disorder.

*Source:* International Classification of Sleep Disorders, Second Edition: Diagnostic and Coding Manual. American Academy of Sleep Medicine. 2006.

## Sleep-related breathing disorders

The disorders in this subgroup are characterized by disordered respiration during sleep. Central sleep apnea syndromes include those in which respiratory effort is diminished or absent in an intermittent or cyclical fashion due to central nervous system or cardiac dysfunction. The obstructive sleep apnea syndromes include those in which there is an obstruction in the airway resulting in continued breathing effort but inadequate ventilation.[3]

There are five major categories of SRBD: central sleep apnea (CSA), obstructive sleep apnea (OSA), sleep-related hypoventilation/hypoxemia, sleep-related hypoventilation/hypoxemia due to medical condition, and other SRBD (unspecified). Only CSA and OSA will be discussed.

### Central sleep apnea syndromes

Characterisic of CSA is the absence of airflow and ventilatory effort for at least 10 seconds during sleep. Although the etiology is unknown, there are investigations suggesting that this disorder is related to cardiac problems or central nervous system dysfunction associated with a ventilatory controller mechanism.[18,19] There may also be an airway collapse, but this is not necessarily a diagnostic event.[20] A PSG in the sleep laboratory similar to the evaluation for OSA is necessary for diagnosis. However, different than the PSG demonstrating OSA, there is an absence of any respiratory effort throughout the duration of the apneic episode for CSA.[21]

There are five types of CSA syndromes (Table 3.1), four of which are further defined here.

**Table 3.8**  *ICSD-2* diagnostic criteria for primary central sleep apnea.

A.  The patient reports at least one of the following:
    a.  Excessive daytime sleepiness
    b.  Frequent arousals and awakenings during sleep or insomnia complaints
    c.  Awakening short of breath.
B.  Polysomnography shows five or more central apneas per hour of sleep.
C.  The disorder is not better explained by another current sleep disorder, medical or neurological disorder, medication use, or substance use disorder.

*Source:* International Classification of Sleep Disorders, Second Edition: Diagnostic and Coding Manual. American Academy of Sleep Medicine. 2006.

### Primary central sleep apnea

Primary central sleep apnea is of unknown etiology and is characterized on the PSG by recurrent cessation of respiration during sleep with the apnea having no associated ventilator effort.[3]

The absence of airflow and respiratory effort is characteristic of primary CSA, and five or more of these types of apneic events per hour are needed to be demonstrated on the PSG. Clinically, the patient will typically present with symptoms of insomnia and EDS or fatigue, and sometimes difficulty with breathing while sleeping, such as awakening with choking (Table 3.8).

### Cheyne–Stokes breathing pattern

Cheyne–Stokes breathing pattern is characterized by recurrent apneas, hypopneas, or both apneas and hypopneas alternating with prolonged hyperpneas during which tidal volume gradually waxes and wanes in a crescendo–decrescendo pattern.[3]

Characteristics for CSA due to Cheyne–Stokes breathing pattern are repeated apneas that alternate with prolonged episodes of hyperpnea, that is deep and rapid respiratory efforts.[22,23] Although Cheyne–Stokes breathing (Figure 3.1) can occur during sleep or waking hours, this abnormal breathing pattern is an indication of a more advanced disorder, such as congestive heart failure, when it does occur during waking hours (Table 3.9).

### High-altitude periodic breathing

High-altitude periodic breathing is characterized by cycling periods of apnea and hyperpnea with the apnea being associated with no ventilator effort (a central apnea).[3]

Characteristic for high-altitude periodic breathing is a sleep disorder caused by an acute mountain sickness.[24] Typically, this will occur when sleeping at altitudes higher than 15,000 feet, especially when not adapted to that altitude (Table 3.10).

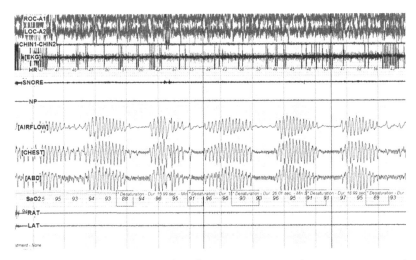

**Figure 3.1**    Cheyne–Stokes breathing pattern. Note characteristic crescendo and decrescendo pattern in breathing effort, paralleling the airflow. (Kakkar R and Hill G. Interpretation of the adult polysomnogram. Otolaryngol Clin North Am. 2007; 40(3):736. Reprinted with permission.)

**Table 3.9**    *ICSD-2 diagnostic criteria for Cheyne–Stokes breathing pattern.*

---

A.    Polysomnography shows at least ten central apneas and hypopneas per hour of sleep in which the hypopnea has a crescendo–decrescendo pattern of tidal volume accompanied by frequent arousals from sleep and derangement of sleep structure.

*NOTE:* Although symptoms are not mandatory to make this diagnosis, patients often report excessive daytime sleepiness, frequent arousals and awakenings during sleep, insomnia complaints, or awakening short of breath.

B.    The breathing disorder occurs in association with a serious medical illness, such as heart failure, stroke, or renal failure.

C.    The disorder is not better explained by another current sleep disorder, medication use, or substance use disorder.

---

*Source:* International Classification of Sleep Disorders, Second Edition: Diagnostic and Coding Manual. American Academy of Sleep Medicine. 2006.

**Table 3.10**    *ICSD-2 diagnostic criteria for high-altitude periodic breathing.*

---

A.    Recent ascent to altitude of at least 4,000 meters.

B.    Polysomnography demonstrates recurrent central apneas, primarily during nonrapid eye movement (NREM) sleep at a frequency greater than 5 per hour. The cycle length should be 12 to 34 seconds.

*NOTE:* Because high-altitude periodic breathing is a normal adaptation to altitude, there are no specific criteria regarding the frequency of central apneas that should be considered normal or abnormal. Although no specific symptoms are required, recurrent awakening during the night and fatigue during the day may be present.

---

*Source:* International Classification of Sleep Disorders, Second Edition: Diagnostic and Coding Manual. American Academy of Sleep Medicine. 2006.

**Table 3.11**   *ICSD-2* diagnostic criteria for central sleep apnea due to drug or substance.

| | |
|---|---|
| A. | The patient has been taking a long-acting opioid regularly for at least 2 months. |
| B. | Polysomnography shows a central apnea index of 5 or more periodic breathing (ten or more central apneas and hypopneas per hour of sleep in which the hypopnea has a crescendo–decrescendo pattern of tidal volume, accompanied by frequent arousals from sleep and derangement of sleep structure). |
| C. | The disorder is not better explained by another current sleep disorder or medical or neurological disorder. |

*Source:* International Classification of Sleep Disorders, Second Edition: Diagnostic and Coding Manual. American Academy of Sleep Medicine. 2006.

## Central sleep apnea due to drug or substance

A small number of studies have documented that users of long-acting opioids may have central apneas during sleep.[3]

This type of CSA is caused by substance or drug use, usually the long-acting opioid pain medications, such as methadone and hydrocodone, with the former being the major contributor (Table 3.11).[25,26]

## *Obstructive sleep apnea syndromes*

Obstructive sleep apnea (OSA) is characterized by repetitive episodes of complete (apnea) or partial (hypopnea) upper airway obstruction occurring during sleep.[3]

Sleep apnea literally involves the cessation of breathing on a repeated basis during sleep. This can occur for a brief period of time for a few seconds to longer than a minute, and the frequency can be as much as several hundreds of times during a sleep period.

OSA typically involves an airway obstruction that results in an increased respiratory effort and insufficient ventilation. OSA can involve complete blockage of the upper airway resulting in an apneic episode or partial blockage of the airway resulting in a hypopneic episode.[27–29] Whereas apnea is complete cessation of airflow, hypopnea is characterized by a 70% reduction of airflow for $\geq$10 seconds or any reduction in airflow that is associated with either an arousal from sleep or a $\geq$3% arterial oxygen desaturation.[30] Apneas and hypopneas as a result of these varying degrees and locations of upper airway obstructions are regarded as the most common SRBD.[31]

As measured by pulse oximetry, associated with these episodes are reduced blood oxygen saturation in spite of inspiratory efforts. Also associated is sleep fragmentation or disruption of the quality and duration of sleep along with the possible subjective reports of EDS and/or insomnia because of the repetitive arousals or awakenings that occur in an effort to

**Table 3.12** *ICSD-2* diagnostic criteria for obstructive sleep apnea, adult.

*NOTE:* A, B, and D or C and D satisfy the criteria.

A.  At least one of the following applies:
    a.  The patient complains of unintentional sleep episodes during wakefulness, daytime sleepiness, unrefreshing sleep, fatigue, or insomnia
    b.  The patient wakes with breath holding, gasping, or choking
    c.  The bed partner reports loud snoring, breathing interruptions, or both during the patient's sleep.
B.  Polysomnographic recording the following:
    a.  Five or more scoreable respiratory events (i.e., apneas, hypopneas, or respiratory effort-related arousals (RERAs)) per hour of sleep
    b.  Evidence of respiratory effort during all or a portion of each respiratory event (in the case of an RERA, this is best seen with the use of esophageal manometry).

**OR**

C.  Polysomnographic recording the following:
    a.  Fifteen or more scoreable respiratory events (i.e., apneas, hypopneas, or RERAs) per hour of sleep
    b.  Evidence of respiratory effort during all or a portion of each respiratory event (in the case of an RERA, this is best seen with the use of esophageal manometry).
D.  The disorder is not better explained by another current sleep disorder, medical or neurological disorder, medication use, or substance use disorder.

*Source:* International Classification of Sleep Disorders, Second Edition: Diagnostic and Coding Manual. American Academy of Sleep Medicine. 2006.

establish airway patency. In order for a diagnosis of OSA to be made, a sleep study must demonstrate a minimum of five or more apenic or hypopneic episodes per each hour of sleep or 30 episodes per 6 hours of sleep.[32] Although obstruction of the upper airway may include multiple anatomical sites, closure of the upper airway is most commonly located in the retropalatal and retroglossal areas (Table 3.12).[33–35]

## Hypersomnias of central origin (not due to a circadian rhythm sleep disorder, SRBD, or other cause of disturbed nocturnal sleep)

This section includes a group of disorders in which the primary complaint is daytime sleepiness and in which the cause of the primary symptom is not disturbed nocturnal sleep or misaligned circadian rhythms.[3]

EDS is regarded as sleepiness that interferes with activities and quality of life during the waking hours. The individual is typically unable to remain alert and awake during the hours that are normally regarded as the waking hours for that individual. EDS may be an indication that the individual is suffering from an inadequate amount of sleep, a fragmented or disrupted sleep, or a sleep disorder.

The *ICSD-2* defines daytime sleepiness, or hypersomnia, as "the inability to stay awake and alert during the major waking episodes of the day, resulting in unintended lapses into drowsiness or sleep."[3] Specifically, hypersomnias of central origin are not caused by SRBD, circadian rhythm sleep disorder, or other causes of disturbed nocturnal sleep. The two more common ones are discussed here.

### Narcolepsy with cataplexy

Narcolepsy with cataplexy is primarily characterized by excessive daytime sleepiness and cataplexy. Many of the symptoms of narcolepsy with cataplexy are due to an unusual proclivity to transition rapidly from wakefulness into rapid eye movement (REM) sleep and to experience dissociated REM sleep events (Table 3.13).[3]

### Narcolepsy without cataplexy

Excessive daytime sleepiness in narcolepsy without cataplexy is most typically associated with naps that are refreshing in nature while nocturnal sleep is normal or moderately disturbed without excessive amounts of sleep (Table 3.14).[3]

The two most common types of narcolepsy are *narcolepsy with cataplexy* and *narcolepsy without cataplexy*.[36,37] Cataplexy is regarded as a sudden but transient loss of muscle tone that is typically triggered by emotions. Some individuals who initially do not exhibit cataplexy will subsequently develop such episodes with their narcolepsy.[3]

The Multiple Sleep Latency Test (MSLT) is used to assess daytime sleepiness and diagnose narcolepsy.[38,39]

## Circadian rhythm sleep disorder

For optimal sleep, the desired sleep time should match the timing of the circadian rhythm of sleep and wake propensity. Therefore, a recurrent or chronic pattern of sleep disturbance may result from alterations of the circadian timing system or a misalignment between the timing of the individual's circadian rhythm of sleep propensity and the 24-hour social and physical environments.[3]

**Table 3.13** *ICSD-2* diagnostic criteria for narcolepsy with cataplexy.

A.  The patient has a complaint of excessive daytime sleepiness occurring almost daily for at least 3 months.
B.  A definite history of cataplexy, defined as sudden and transient episodes of loss of muscle tone triggered by emotions, is present.

*NOTE:* To be labeled as cataplexy, these episodes must be triggered by strong emotions—most reliably laughing or joking—and must be generally bilateral and brief (less than 2 minutes). Consciousness is preserved, at least at the beginning of the episode. Observed cataplexy with transient reversible loss of deep tendon reflexes is a very strong, but rare, diagnostic finding.

C.  The diagnosis of narcolepsy with cataplexy should, whenever possible, be confirmed by nocturnal polysomnography followed by a Multiple Sleep Latency Test (MSLT); the mean sleep latency on MSLT is less than or equal to 8 minutes and two or more sleep onset REM periods (SOREMPs) are observed following sufficient nocturnal sleep (minimum 6 hours) during the night prior to the test. Alternatively, hypocretin-1 levels in the cerebospinal fluid (CSF) are less than or equal to 110 pg/mL or one-third of mean normal control values.

*NOTE:* The presence of one or more SOREMPs during the MSLT is a very specific finding, whereas a mean sleep latency of less than 8 minutes can be found in up to 30% of the normal population. Low CSF hypocretin-1 levels (less than or equal to 110 pg/mL or one-third of mean normal control values) are found in more than 90% of patients with narcolepsy with cataplexy and almost never in controls or in other patients with other pathologies.

D.  The hypersomnia is not better explained by another sleep disorder, medical or neurological disorder, mental disorder, medication use, or substance use disorder.

*Source:* International Classification of Sleep Disorders, Second Edition: Diagnostic and Coding Manual. American Academy of Sleep Medicine. 2006.

**Table 3.14** *ICSD-2* diagnostic criteria for narcolepsy without cataplexy.

A.  The patient has a complaint of excessive daytime sleepiness occurring almost daily for at least 3 months.
B.  Typical cataplexy is not present, although doubtful or atypical cataplexy-like episodes may be reported.
C.  The diagnosis of narcolepsy without cataplexy must be confirmed by nocturnal polysomnography followed by an Multiple Sleep Latency Test (MSLT). In narcolepsy without cataplexy, the mean sleep latency on MSLT is less than or equal to 8 minutes and two or more SOREMPs are observed following sufficient nocturnal sleep (minimum 6 hours) during the night prior to the test.

*NOTE:* The presence of two or more SOREMPs during the MSLT is a very specific finding, whereas a mean sleep latency of less than 8 minutes can be found in up to 30% of the normal population.

D.  The hypersomnia is not better explained by another sleep disorder, medical or neurological disorder, mental disorder, medication use, or substance use disorder.

*Source:* International Classification of Sleep Disorders, Second Edition: Diagnostic and Coding Manual. American Academy of Sleep Medicine. 2006.

**Table 3.15** *ICSD-2* general criteria for circadian rhythm sleep disorders.

| | |
|---|---|
| A. | There is a persistent or recurrent pattern of sleep disturbance due primarily to one of the following: |
| | a.  Alterations of the circadian timekeeping system |
| | b.  Misalignment between the endogenous circadian rhythm and exogenous factors that affect the timing or duration of sleep. |
| B. | The circadian-related sleep disruption leads to insomnia, excessive daytime sleepiness, or both. |
| C. | The sleep disturbance is associated with impairment of social, occupational, or other areas of functioning. |

*Source:* International Classification of Sleep Disorders, Second Edition: Diagnostic and Coding Manual. American Academy of Sleep Medicine. 2006.

Circadian rhythm sleep disorders (CRSD) should be included as a possibility when considering a differential diagnosis of individuals who report EDS, insomnia, and impairment of daily functional activities.

Circadian in Latin means "about a day." The human body has an internal timing that demonstrates a circadian rhythm, and one of the more powerful external stimuli for indicating time is the light–dark cycle.[40] Another time indicator for the body is melatonin, which is low during the day since light suppresses the secretion of melatonin and increases as the body prepares for the onset of sleep.[41]

The common chronophysiologic characteristic of CRSD is the recurrent asynchrony between the individual's pattern of sleep and what is regarded as society's norm for sleep.[40,42] With most CRSD cases, the individual has difficulty sleeping at the desired sleep time or when it is required. When there is the desynchronization of the individual's circadian clock relative to the light–dark cycle, CRSD can occur (Table 3.15).[3]

There are nine recognized types of CRSD in the *ICSD-2*, but two of the more common are discussed here.

## Jet lag type

Circadian rhythm sleep disorder, jet lag type, is a circadian rhythm sleep disorder in which there is a temporary mismatch between the timing of the sleep and wake cycle generated by the endogenous circadian clock and that of the sleep and wake pattern required by a change in time zone.[3]

Jet lag type (jet lag sleep disorder) occurs when there is a transient misalignment of the individual's internal circadian sleep–wake cycle and the new time zone associated with the external environment. Typically, this type of CRSD worsens in relation to the number of crossed time zones.[43] Individuals with jet lag sleep disorder typically report a history of difficulty falling asleep at the desired time as well as EDS during the waking

**Table 3.16**  *ICSD-2* diagnostic criteria for circadian rhythm disorder, jet lag type.

A.  There is a complaint of insomnia or excessive daytime sleepiness associated with transmeridian jet travel across at least two time zones.
B.  There is associated impairment of daytime function, general malaise, or somatic symptoms such as gastrointestinal disturbance within 1 or 2 days after travel.
C.  The sleep disturbance is not better explained by another current sleep disorder, medical or neurological disorder, mental disorder, medication use, or substance use disorder.

*Source:* International Classification of Sleep Disorders, Second Edition: Diagnostic and Coding Manual. American Academy of Sleep Medicine. 2006.

hours. It is not uncommon to have disturbed sleep and impaired function during the waking hours associated with this disorder (Table 3.16).

## Shift work type

Circadian rhythm sleep disorder, shift work type, is characterized by complaints of insomnia or excessive sleepiness that occur in relation to work hours that are scheduled during the usual sleep period.[3]

Shift work type (shift work sleep disorder) features insomnia or EDS that is associated with the scheduling of an individual's hours of work during the usual times for sleep for that individual. This type of time shift typically includes night shifts, early morning shifts, or rotating shifts. The adverse affect on sleep quality can result in EDS, insomnia, impaired function during the waking hours, and increased irritability.[44,45] Specifically, these individuals will report a history of insomnia during their scheduled sleep time as well as EDS during their scheduled work time (Table 3.17).

**Table 3.17**  *ICSD-2* diagnostic criteria for circadian rhythm disorder, shift work type.

A.  There is a complaint of insomnia or excessive daytime sleepiness associated with a recurring work schedule that overlaps the usual time for sleep.
B.  The symptoms are associated with the shift work schedule over the course of at least 1 month.
C.  Sleep log or actigraphy monitoring (with sleep diaries) for at least 7 days demonstrates disturbed circadian and sleep time misalignment.
D.  The sleep disturbance is not better explained by another current sleep disorder, medical or neurological disorder, mental disorder, medication use, or substance use disorder.

*Source:* International Classification of Sleep Disorders, Second Edition: Diagnostic and Coding Manual. American Academy of Sleep Medicine. 2006.

# Parasomnias

Parasomnias are undesirable physical events or experiences that occur during entry into sleep, within sleep, or during arousals from sleep.[3]

Parasomnias are undesirable and unintentional physical and/or subjective experiences that occur as the individual begins to enter into sleep, during sleep, or during arousals from sleep.[3,46-49] Included in these disorders are sleep-related movements, emotions, behaviors, dreaming, and functioning of the autonomic nervous system. Parasomnias often take place during arousal and transitions between sleep states when there is reorganization of brain activity, which lends to the belief that the sleep and waking states are not mutually exclusive. The result, therefore, of the overlap of one state with the other results in parasomnias.[49,50]

Of the parasomnias, those considered to be disorders of arousal are the most common and can manifest in 4% of the adult population.[51] Examples of such arousals can include sleepwalking, mumbling, shrieking, disorientation upon awakening, limb paralysis, and uncontrollable eating.[52]

The more common of the parasomnias will be discussed here.

## Confusional arousals

Confusional arousals consist of mental confusion or confusional behavior during or following arousals from sleep, typically from slow-wave sleep in the first part of the night, but also upon attempted awakening from sleep in the morning.[3]

Characteristic of confusional arousals is the display of confused or disoriented mental and behavior activities that can take place during and after awakening from sleep.[3] Although this disorder is most common in younger children, it can occur with adults (Table 3.18).

## Sleepwalking

Sleepwalking consists of a series of complex behaviors that are usually initiated during arousals from slow-wave sleep and culminate in walking around with an altered state of consciousness and impaired judgment.[3]

**Table 3.18** *ICSD-2 diagnostic criteria for confusional arousals.*

| | |
|---|---|
| A. | Recurrent mental confusion or confusional behavior occurs during an arousal or awakening from nocturnal sleep or a daytime nap. |
| B. | The disturbance is not better explained by another sleep disorder, medical or neurological disorder, mental disorder, medication use, or substance use disorder. |

*Source:* International Classification of Sleep Disorders, Second Edition: Diagnostic and Coding Manual. American Academy of Sleep Medicine. 2006.

**Table 3.19** *ICSD-2* diagnostic criteria for sleepwalking.

A.  Ambulation occurs during sleep.
B.  Persistence of sleep, an altered state of consciousness, or impaired judgment during ambulation is demonstrated by at least one of the following:
    a.  Difficulty in arousing the person
    b.  Mental confusion when awakened from an episode
    c.  Amnesia (complete or partial) for the episode
    d.  Routine behaviors that occur at inappropriate times
    e.  Inappropriate or nonsensical behaviors
    f.  Dangerous or potentially dangerous behaviors.
C.  The disturbance is not better explained by another sleep disorder, medical or neurological disorder, mental disorder, medication use, or substance use disorder.

*Source:* International Classification of Sleep Disorders, Second Edition: Diagnostic and Coding Manual. American Academy of Sleep Medicine. 2006.

Sleepwalking, also known as somnambulism, is characterized by walking behavior during an altered state of consciousness and impaired judgment.[3] However, sleepwalking can also involve simply sitting up in one's bed. Inappropriate behavior, such as urinating in the middle of a room, can occur during sleepwalking, and even injuries can occur (e.g., falling down a set of stairs) which may cause trauma to the maxillomandibular region. Typically, these individuals do not remember sleepwalking occurrences (Table 3.19).

### Sleep terrors

Sleep terrors consist of arousals from slow-wave sleep accompanied by a cry or piercing scream and autonomic nervous system and behavioral manifestations of intense fear.[3]

Sleep terrors are considered to be the most dramatic of the arousal disorders since it is common for the individual to exhibit screaming or crying along with extreme panic.[3] There are usually autonomic system responses, such as tachycardia and increased muscle tone, along with intense fear. When these events occur, the individual typically sits up in bed and can even display significant motor activity that can include hitting walls and running around or even out of a bedroom,[49] again with the potential to cause physical injury such as trauma to the maxillomandibular region. The individual can be difficult to awaken, and upon awakening from an episode, the individual is usually confused and does not remember the episode (Table 3.20).

### Recurrent isolated sleep paralysis

Recurrent isolated sleep paralysis is characterized by an inability to perform voluntary movements at sleep onset (hypnagogic or predormital form) or on waking from sleep (hypnopompic or postdormital form) in the absence of a diagnosis of narcolepsy.[3]

**Table 3.20** *ICSD-2* diagnostic criteria for sleep terrors.

A.  A sudden episode of terror occurs during sleep, usually initiated by a cry or
    loud scream that is accompanied by autonomic nervous system and behavioral
    manifestations of intense fear.
B.  At least one of the following associated features is present:
    a.  Difficulty in arousing the person
    b.  Mental confusion when awakened from an episode
    c.  Amnesia (complete or partial) for the episode
    d.  Dangerous or potentially dangerous behaviors.
C.  The disturbance is not better explained by another sleep disorder, medical or
    neurological disorder, mental disorder, medication use, or substance use
    disorder.

*Source:* International Classification of Sleep Disorders, Second Edition: Diagnostic and Coding
Manual. American Academy of Sleep Medicine. 2006.

Recurrent isolated sleep paralysis features an individual's inability to
perform voluntary motor function of the limbs, trunk, and head at the time
of onset of sleep or upon awakening. Typically, respiratory movements are
not affected and cognition is not impaired. It is not uncommon for there to
be associated hallucinations.

This type of disorder can have episodes with a duration of 1 to several
minutes. Individuals have indicated such events to be extremely frightening (Table 3.21).

## Nightmare disorder

Nightmare disorder is characterized by recurrent nightmares,
which are disturbing mental experiences that generally occur during REM sleep and that often result in awakening.[3]

Nightmare disorder is characterized by dream patterns and themes that
are increasingly frightening or distressing during the sleep period such that

**Table 3.21** *ICSD-2* diagnostic criteria for sleep paralysis.

A.  The patient complains of an inability to move the trunk and all limbs at sleep
    onset or on waking from sleep.
B.  Each episode lasts seconds to a few minutes.
C.  The disturbance is not better explained by another sleep disorder (particularly
    narcolepsy), a medical or neurological disorder, mental disorder, medication
    use, or substance use disorder.
*NOTE:* Hallucinatory experiences may be present but are not essential to the
diagnosis. Polysomnography, if performed, reveals the event to occur at a
dissociated state with elements of rapid eye movement (REM) sleep and wakefulness.

*Source:* International Classification of Sleep Disorders, Second Edition: Diagnostic and Coding
Manual. American Academy of Sleep Medicine. 2006.

**Table 3.22** *ICSD-2* diagnostic criteria for nightmare disorder.

A.   Recurrent episodes of awakenings from sleep with recall of intensely disturbing dream mentation, usually involving fear or anxiety, but also anger, sadness, disgust, and other dysphoric emotions.
B.   Full alertness on awakening, with little confusion or disorientation; recall of sleep mentation is immediate and clear.
C.   At least one of the following associated features is present:
    a.   Delayed return to sleep after the episodes
    b.   Occurrence of episodes in the latter half of the habitual sleep period.

*Source:* International Classification of Sleep Disorders, Second Edition: Diagnostic and Coding Manual. American Academy of Sleep Medicine. 2006.

the individual can awaken with intense fear and anxiety. Usually this disorder is accompanied by an increase in heart and respiratory rates.[53] Individuals have indicated that it can be difficult to return to sleep after such an episode (Table 3.22).

## Sleep-related eating disorder

Sleep related eating disorder (SRED) consists of recurrent episodes of involuntary eating and drinking during arousals from sleep with problematic consequences.[3]

Sleep-related eating disorder is characterized by repeated episodes of eating and/or drinking during arousals or partial arousals from sleep. This type of disorder may result in trauma to the maxillomandibular region, such as tongue biting or tooth fracture. Typically, this disorder involves an uncontrollable behavior of which the individual does not recall upon awakening (Table 3.23).

# Sleep-related movement disorders

Sleep-related movement disorders are conditions that are primarily characterized by relatively simple, usually stereotyped, movements that disturb sleep or by other sleep-related monophasic movement disorders such as sleep-related leg cramps.[3]

Sleep-related movement disorders constitute characteristic body movements that cause sleep disturbance. The most common ones are discussed here.

## Restless legs syndrome

Restless legs syndrome (RLS) is a sensorimotor disorder characterized by a complaint of a strong, nearly irresistible, urge to move the legs. This urge to move is often but not always accompanied by other uncomfortable paresthesias felt deep inside the legs or as a feeling that is simply difficult or impossible to describe.[3]

**Table 3.23**  *ICSD-2 diagnostic criteria for sleep-related eating disorder.*

A.  Recurrent episodes of involuntary eating and drinking occur during the main sleep period.
B.  One or more of the following must be present with the recurrent episodes of involuntary eating and drinking:
    a.  Consumption of peculiar forms or combinations of food or inedible or toxic substances
    b.  Insomnia related to sleep disruption from repeated episodes of eating, with a complaint of nonrestorative sleep, daytime fatigue, or somnolence
    c.  Sleep-related injury
    d.  Dangerous behaviors performed while in pursuit of food or while cooking food
    e.  Morning anorexia
    f.  Adverse health consequences from recurring binge eating of high caloric foods.
C.  The disturbance is not better explained by another sleep disorder, medical or neurological disorder, mental disorder, medication use, or substance use disorder.

*Source:* International Classification of Sleep Disorders, Second Edition: Diagnostic and Coding Manual. American Academy of Sleep Medicine. 2006.

Episodes of RLS are present mainly when the individual is at rest or during periods of inactivity, and they occur later in the day/evening or as the individual is attempting to initiate sleep.[54] Generally, the experience can have a duration of a few minutes to several hours.

Individuals often describe associated paresthesias or uncomfortable sensations such as jittery or itchy feelings being associated with RLS. The urge to move the legs and the paresthesias can be so unpleasant as to preclude the individual from initiating asleep.[55] It has also been reported that individuals can awaken from sleep because of the RLS episode.[56] Often the individual will relieve these sensations by getting up and walking.[57,58] It is not uncommon to associate RLS in individuals who demonstrate reduced iron levels along with renal failure (Table 3.24).[59,60,61]

## Periodic limb movement disorder

Periodic limb movement disorder (PLMD) is characterized by periodic episodes of repetitive, highly stereotyped, limb movements that occur during sleep (PLMS) and by clinical sleep disturbance that cannot be accounted for by another primary sleep disorder.[3]

Periodic limb movement disorder (PLMD) is characterized by repetitive limb movements that occur during sleep.[62] PLMD can be associated with RLS, although PLMD can stand alone as episode independent of RLS. These periodic episodes of limb movement can result in sleep disturbances,[3] although the individual is usually unaware of such partial

**Table 3.24**  *ICSD-2* diagnostic criteria for restless legs syndrome for adults.

A.  The patient reports an urge to move the legs, usually accompanied or caused by uncomfortable and unpleasant sensations in the legs.

B.  The urge to move or the unpleasant sensations begin or worsen during periods of rest or inactivity such as lying or sitting.

C.  The urge to move or the unpleasant sensations are partially or totally relieved by movement, such as walking or stretching, at least as long as the activity continues.

D.  The urge to move or the unpleasant sensations are worse, or only occur, in the evening or night.

E.  The condition is not better explained by another current sleep disorder, medical or neurological disorder, mental disorder, medication use, or substance use disorder.

*Source:* International Classification of Sleep Disorders, Second Edition: Diagnostic and Coding Manual. American Academy of Sleep Medicine. 2006.

arousal or awakenings. Even though the disorder is unrecognized by the individual, it is not uncommon for the individual to report a history of EDS and/or insomnia.

PLMD usually displays as extensions of the big toe or flexions of the ankle, knee, or hip,[63] but it can also involve the upper limbs (Table 3.25).

## Sleep-related leg cramps

Sleep-related leg cramps are painful sensations caused by sudden and intense involuntary contractions of muscles or muscle groups, usually in the calf of small muscles of the foot, occurring during the sleep period.[3]

Sleep-related leg cramps are characterized by sudden intense muscle contractions that occur during sleep. Typically, the muscles of the calves or feet are affected. This disorder has also been known as "Charley Horse."

These cramps usually occur during sleep, which then result in a disruption of sleep such as an arousal or even an awakening with severe pain. Because of these disruptions to sleep, the individual may report EDS and/or insomnia (Table 3.26).

## Sleep-related bruxism

Sleep-related bruxism is an oral activity characterized by grinding or clenching of the teeth during sleep, usually associated with sleep arousals.[3]

Sleep-related bruxism (SRB) is an oromotor activity characterized by clenching and/or grinding of the teeth during sleep, and it is regarded as a separate entity than bruxism that occurs during the waking hours.[64,65]

**Table 3.25** *ICSD-2 diagnostic criteria for periodic limb movement disorder.*

A. Polysomnography demonstrates repetitive, highly stereotyped limb movements that are
   a. 0.5–5 seconds in duration
   b. Of amplitude greater than or equal to 25% of toe dorsiflexion during calibration
   c. In a sequence of four or more movements
   d. Separated by an interval of more than 5 seconds (from limb-movement onset to limb-movement onset) and less than 90 seconds (typically there is an interval of 20–40 seconds).
B. The PLMS index exceeds 5 per hour in children and 15 per hour in most adult cases.

*NOTE:* The PLMS index must be interpreted in the context of a patient's sleep-related complaint. In adults, normative values higher than the previously accepted value of 5 per hour have been found in studies that did not exclude respiratory event-related arousals (using sensitive respiratory monitoring) and other causes for PLMS. New data suggest a partial overlap of PLMS index values between symptomatic and asymptomatic individuals, emphasizing the importance of clinical context over an absolute cutoff value.
C. There is clinical sleep disturbance or a complaint of daytime fatigue.

*NOTE:* If PLMS are present without clinical sleep disturbance, the PLMS can be noted as a polysomnographic finding, but criteria are not met for a diagnosis of PLMD.
D. The PLMs are not better explained by another current sleep disorder, medical or neurological disorder, mental disorder, medication use, or substance use disorder (e.g., PLMs at the termination of cyclically occurring apneas should not be counted as true PLMS or PLMD).

*Source:* International Classification of Sleep Disorders, Second Edition: Diagnostic and Coding Manual. American Academy of Sleep Medicine. 2006.

In dentistry, bruxism is regarded as a mandibular parafunctional activity, whereas in sleep medicine, SRB is considered to be a movement disorder. Because of this difference, SRB is included in the *ICSD-2* category of sleep-related movement disorders.

**Table 3.26** *ICSD-2 diagnostic criteria for sleep-related leg cramps.*

A. A painful sensation in the leg or foot is associated with sudden muscle hardness or tightness indicating a strong muscle contraction.
B. The painful muscle contractions in the legs or feet occur during the sleep period, although they may arise from either wakefulness or sleep.
C. The pain is relieved by forceful stretching of the affected muscles, releasing the contraction.
D. The sleep-related leg cramps are not better explained by another current sleep disorder, medical or neurological disorder, mental disorder, medication use, or substance use disorder.

*Source:* International Classification of Sleep Disorders, Second Edition: Diagnostic and Coding Manual. American Academy of Sleep Medicine. 2006.

**Table 3.27**  *ICSD-2* diagnostic criteria for sleep-related bruxism.

A.  The patient reports or is aware of tooth-grinding sounds or tooth clenching during sleep.
B.  One or more of the following is present:
    a.  Abnormal wear of the teeth
    b.  Jaw muscle discomfort, fatigue, or pain and jaw lock upon awakening
    c.  Masseter muscle hypertrophy upon voluntary forceful clenching.
C.  The jaw muscle activity is not better explained by another current sleep disorder, medical or neurological disorder, mental disorder, medication use, or substance use disorder.

*Source:* International Classification of Sleep Disorders, Second Edition: Diagnostic and Coding Manual. American Academy of Sleep Medicine. 2006.

In addition to creating noise that may disturb the sleep of the bed partner, these involuntary mandibular movement episodes may cause arousals during the sleep period as well as abrasion wear of the teeth and restorations, changes of the periodontal tissues, hypersensitivity of the dentition, masticatory myalgia, and restriction of mandibular movement. Along with the studies demonstrating the relationship that emotional stress and psychosocial factors can have with SRBD,[66,67] the microarousal effect of this activity on sleep architecture has been shown to be associated with the central and autonomic nervous system processes.[68] In addition, individuals with SRBD have been shown to have more frequent body movements when compared to individuals without SRBD (Table 3.27).[69]

## Isolated symptoms, apparently normal variants and unresolved issues

Sleep-related symptoms that either lie at the borderline between normal and abnormal sleep or that exist on the continuum of normal to abnormal events in sleep are included in this section.[3]

### Snoring

Snoring is a respiratory sound generated in the upper airway during sleep that typically occurs during inspiration but may also occur in expiration; the snoring described here occurs without episodes of apnea or hypoventilation.[3]

The *Merriam-Webster Online Dictionary* defines snoring as "to breathe during sleep with a rough hoarse noise due to vibration of the soft palate."[70] The resultant noise involves a vibration interaction of the airflow with the muscles and pharyngeal walls of the upper airway, particularly in the areas of the soft palate, uvula, and pharyngeal airway. Snoring is more often observed during inspiration, but it can also occur during expiration.

Snoring is very common with an occurrence in 24% of adult females and 40% of adult males.[71] Because snoring is usually more of a complaint for the bed partner than it is for the snorer, the noise is typically the primary reason for seeking a medical consult. Not all individuals who snore have OSA, but those individuals with OSA generally demonstrate a snoring component during their sleep period.[72] Thus, it is possible for snoring to be a precursor to OSA.

When snoring occurs without any sleep pattern fragmentation or respiratory apneic or hypopneic episodes, it is often referred to as primary (benign) snoring.[2,73,74] Whereas individuals with OSA will report the classic descriptions of EDS or insomnia, individuals with primary or benign snoring will not have these experiences.[73,75] However, snoring may also be associated with many of the same symptoms as OSA.

Unfortunately, the individual who snores may not be aware of the association of OSA symptoms and snoring, and thus some snorers may also experience EDS along with associated but underlying subclinical health issues that have not been brought to the attention of his or her primary care physician (Table 3.28).[76–83]

## Other sleep disorders

Those sleep disorders that cannot be classified elsewhere in the *ICSD-2* are listed in this category. There are several reasons why a sleep disorder may be classified in this section: 1) the sleep disorder may overlap many other categories, 2) there may be insufficient data collected to firmly establish another diagnosis, 3) it seems likely that new sleep disorders will be discovered during the lifetime of the *ICSD-2*. Such disorders would be classified here until a permanent diagnosis is established in future editions.[3]

### Environmental sleep disorder

Environmental sleep disorder is a sleep disturbance due to a disturbing environmental factor that causes a complaint of either insomnia or daytime fatigue and somnolence.[3]

**Table 3.28** *ICSD-2* diagnostic criteria for snoring.

A.  Audible snoring noises are reported by an observer.
B.  The patient has no complaints of insomnia, excessive daytime sleepiness, or sleep disruption that are attributable to snoring or airflow limitation.

*NOTE:* Polysomnography is not required for the diagnosis of snoring, but, when performed, demonstrates audio signal peaks via microphone that are confirmed by the attendant technical staff to be snoring. These noises are not associated with airflow limitation, arousals from sleep, oxygen desaturations, or cardiac arrhythmias.

*Source:* International Classification of Sleep Disorders, Second Edition: Diagnostic and Coding Manual. American Academy of Sleep Medicine. 2006.

**Table 3.29**  *ICSD-2* diagnostic criteria for environmental sleep disorder.

A.  The patient complains of insomnia, daytime fatigue, or a parasomnia. In cases in which daytime fatigue is present, the daytime fatigue may occur as a result of the accompanying insomnia or as a result of poor quality of nocturnal sleep.
B.  The complaint is temporarily associated with the introduction of a physically measurable stimulus or environmental circumstances that disturb sleep.
C.  It is the physical properties, rather than the psychological meaning of the environmental factor, that account for the sleep complaint.
D.  The sleep disturbance is not better explained by another sleep disorder, medical or neurological disorder, mental disorder, medication use, or substance use disorder.

*Source:* International Classification of Sleep Disorders, Second Edition: Diagnostic and Coding Manual. American Academy of Sleep Medicine. 2006.

Sleep can be disturbed to varying degrees by different environmental factors, including sound, light, temperature, bed partner's snoring and/or OSA, bed motion, and even the psychological factor of needing to maintain an alertness level that may be needed when caring for someone in the household such as an infant.

The prevalence of this disorder is not known, but the practitioner can query the patient about the more common environmental factors that may interfere with sleep. Sometimes it may be necessary to ask the patient to maintain a sleep diary so that patterns can be discerned. The bed partner can also be helpful in providing resourceful information.

An environmentally controlled sleep study may be necessary for a definitive evaluation. If the environmental issues can be resolved, a reduction or even elimination of the sleep disorder usually follows. Otherwise, there may be symptoms of long-term sleep disturbance, affecting the quality of life of the individual (Table 3.29).[84]

## Appendix A: Sleep disorders associated with conditions classifiable elsewhere

Numerous medical disorders affect sleep or are affected by sleep. This appendix is not designed to list them all. Rather, it lists a small number of medical disorders that may be of particular importance to sleep diagnosticians.[3]

### Fibromyalgia

According to the 1990 American College of Rheumatology consensus criteria, fibromyalgia is characterized by widespread pain of at least 3 months' duration and muscle tenderness, as determined by palpation.[3]

One of the greatest challenges for the dentist is to evaluate and diagnose the orofacial pain complaint. A pain that has an etiology localized and related to the tissues of the oral cavity is generally easier to manage than when the pain does not have an obvious source such as a musculoskeletal pain, which can be more systemic with central nervous system involvement.

Fibromyalgia is a syndrome described by multiple tender point sites and long-standing musculoskeletal pain that is usually diffuse. The criteria for fibromyalgia established by the American College of Rheumatology states that there must be a widespread distribution above and below the waist of musculoskeletal pain occurring for a minimum of 3 months along with 11 or more of the 18 recognized tender points.[85] The prevalence of fibromyalgia is the second most common rheumatological disorder after osteoarthritis.

Many individuals with the fibromyalgia syndrome also experience sleep disturbance that can result in feeling tired, unrefreshed sleep, reduced cognitive function, and early awakening from sleep.[86–88] It has been found that most subjects with fibromyalgia experienced microarousals[87] and an electroencephalographic (EEG) alpha-delta or alpha-NREM anomaly that interrupts the deep Stage 4 NREM restorative level of sleep.[89,90] This EEG anomaly, though, may not be specific to fibromyalgia as it has also been found in individuals who did not have fibromyalgia complaints.[91]

Despite these investigative differences with EEG activity and fibromyalgia, the field of sleep medicine does acknowledge the relationship and affect of fibromyalgia syndrome on sleep (Table 3.30).

## Sleep-related headaches

Sleep-related headaches are a group of unilateral or bilateral headaches of varying severity and duration that occur during sleep or upon awakening from sleep.[3]

**Table 3.30**  *ICSD-2* diagnostic criteria for fibromyalgia.

| | |
|---|---|
| A. | A history of widespread pain is present for at least 3 months. The pain affects the left and right sides of the body, above and below the waist, and the axial skeletal regions (cervical, chest, and upper and lower back). |
| B. | Tenderness, as determined by digital palpation with approximately 4 kg of pressure, is present in at least 11 of 18 specific anatomic sites that are located in the following bilateral areas: subocciput, anterior lower cervical at intertransverse spaces at C5–C7, upper borders of mid-trapezius, supraspinatus, second costochondral junctions of the anterior ribcage, lateral epicondyles, gluteals, greater trochanters, and medial fat pad of the knees. |

*Source:* International Classification of Sleep Disorders, Second Edition: Diagnostic and Coding Manual. American Academy of Sleep Medicine. 2006.

Sleep medicine recognizes the association that may exist for some individuals relative to sleep disorders and various headache disorders, including migraine, cluster, chronic daily, awakening or morning, and tension-type headaches.[92] As compared to the general population, individuals with headaches demonstrate a two- to eightfold greater risk for sleep disorders, and the most common sleep disorder associated with headache subjects is insomnia.[93]

It has been suggested that the neuroanatomy of the hypothalamus and the neurophysiological mechanisms involving the secretions of serotonin and melatonin may be contributory to the comorbidity of sleep disorders and headaches.[92] Relative to cluster headache, melatonin secretion may be impaired in those individuals.[94]

Modifications of sleep hygiene such as sleep loss, sleep disturbance, and even oversleeping have been identified as the most common precipitating factors of migraine and tension-type headaches.[95–98] Studies demonstrated a significant increase in SRBD with cluster headache subjects.[99]

For the practitioner involved with orofacial pain populations, it is important to differentiate the sleep-related headache patients from those patients whose headaches may be of different origin. Even though neuroimaging may rule in or out any structural or infection etiology for headache, there are no pathognomonic PSG findings for each of the different types of headaches (Table 3.31).

While there are no empirically established algorithms to guide clinical practice, there are now at least a few empirically supported tenets. The review suggests: (1) chronic daily headache, and especially "morning headache," is a particular, though nonspecific, indicator for sleep disorders; (2) the identification and management of a primary sleep disorder in the presence of headache may improve or resolve the headache (headache secondary to primary sleep disorder); (3) headache patients exhibit a high incidence of sleep disturbance which might trigger or exacerbate headache; and (4) such primary headache may improve with regulation of sleep. These findings argue for screening and management of sleep disturbance among headache patients.[93]

### Sleep-related gastroesophageal reflux

Sleep-related gastroesophageal reflux is characterized by regurgitation of stomach contents into the esophagus during sleep.[3]

**Table 3.31**  *ICSD-2 diagnostic criterion for sleep-related headaches.*

A. The patient complains of headache during sleep or upon awakening from sleep.

*Source:* International Classification of Sleep Disorders, Second Edition: Diagnostic and Coding Manual. American Academy of Sleep Medicine. 2006.

**Table 3.32** *ICSD-2 diagnostic criteria for sleep-related gastroesophageal reflux.*

Either A and B, or C.

A.  The patient complains of recurrent awakenings from sleep with shortness of breath or heartburn.
B.  At least one of the following:
    a.  A sour bitter taste in the mouth upon awakening form sleep
    b.  Sleep-related coughing or choking
    c.  Awakening from sleep with heartburn.
C.  Polysomnography and esophageal pH monitoring demonstrate gastroesophageal reflux during sleep with associated arousal.
D.  The disturbance is not better explained by another sleep disorder, medical or neurological disorder, mental disorder, medication use, or substance use disorder.

*Source:* International Classification of Sleep Disorders, Second Edition: Diagnostic and Coding Manual. American Academy of Sleep Medicine. 2006.

This sleep disorder may result in a pain that is usually located substernal, but it may also manifest in the area of the throat. Gastroesophageal reflux disease (GERD), also more commonly known by patients as heart burn or acid indigestion, may present the same symptoms as with this sleep disorder. The dentist needs to be aware of this sleep disorder because of the patient who may present with a symptom of throat pain (Table 3.32).

## Sleep-related coronary artery ischemia

Sleep-related coronary artery ischemia is characterized by ischemia of the myocardium that occurs at night, presumably during sleep.[3]

Typically, this particular sleep disorder will present itself with the sensation of pressure or pain in the chest area. However, because the patient may present with a symptom of pain radiating to the mandibular area, the practitioner should be familiar with this particular sleep disorder (Table 3.33).

**Table 3.33** *ICSD-2 diagnostic criterion for coronary artery ischemia.*

A. Sleep-related electrocardiographic features of cardiac ischemia are present (ST segment elevation or ST segment depression).
*NOTE:* Identifiable sleep disorders such as OSA may be present and may be temporally associated with the ST segment depression.

*Source:* International Classification of Sleep Disorders, Second Edition: Diagnostic and Coding Manual. American Academy of Sleep Medicine. 2006.

## CONCLUSION

There are numerous sleep disorders that patients may have. For the practicing dentist, it is beneficial if one is knowledgeable of symptoms that may indicate the risk for a sleep disorder.

It is not necessary for the dentist to determine the specific sleep disorder. More important, it is helpful if the dentist can recognize symptoms that may indicate the need for a more appropriate referral.

## REFERENCES

1. Association of Sleep Disorders Centers. Diagnostic classification of sleep and arousal disorders. Prepared by the Sleep Disorders Classification Committee, Roffwarg HP, Chairman. Sleep. 1979; 2:1–137.
2. Diagnostic Classification Steering Committee of the American Sleep Disorders Association. International Classification of Sleep Disorders: Diagnostic and Coding Manual. Rochester, MN: American Academy of Sleep Medicine. 1990; 195.
3. American Academy of Sleep Medicine. International Classification of Sleep Disorders, Second Edition. Westchester, IL: American Academy of Sleep Medicine. 2005.
4. World Health Organization. International Classification of Diseases (ICD). Available at http://www.who.int/classifications/icd/en/, http://www.who.int/classifications/icd/en/HistoryOfICD.pdf. Accessed 2009.
5. Punjabi NM, Welch D, and Strohl K. Sleep disorders in regional sleep centers: a national cooperative study. Coleman II Study Investigators. Sleep. 2000; 23(4):471–480.
6. Ohayon MM. Epidemiology of insomnia: what we know and what we still need to learn. Sleep Med Rev. 2002; 6(2):97–111.
7. Benca RM. Diagnosis and treatment of chronic insomnia: a review. Psychiatr Serv. 2005; 56(3):332–343.
8. Benca RM, Obermeyer WH, Thisted RA, et al. Sleep and psychiatric disorders: a meta-analysis. Arch Gen Psychiatry. 1992; 49:651–668.
9. Perlis ML, Smith MT, and Pigeon WR. Etiology and pathophysiology of insomnia. In: Kryger MH, Roth T, and Dement WC, eds. Principles and Practice of Sleep Medicine. 4th ed. Philadelphia: Elsevier/Saunders. 2005; 714–725.
10. Hauri PJ and Fischer J. Persistent psychophysiological (learned) insomnia. Sleep. 1986; 9:38–53.
11. Reynolds CF, Taska LS, Sewitch DE, et al. Persistent physchophysiologic insomnia: preliminary research, diagnostic criteria, and EEG sleep data. Am J Psychiatry. 1984; 141:804–805.
12. Haynes SN, Adams A, and Franzen M. The effects of pre-sleep stress on sleep-onset insomnia. J Abnorm Psychol. 1981; 90:601–606.

13. Morin CM, Rodriquez S, and Ivers H. Role of stress, arousal, and coping skills in primary insomnia. Psychosom Med. 2003; 65:259–267.

14. Spielman AJ. Assessment of insomnia. Clin Psychol Rev. 1986; 6:11–25.

15. Morin CM, Hauri PJ, Espie CA, et al. Nonpharmacologic treatment of chronic insomnia. An American Academy of Sleep Medicine review. Sleep. 1986; 22:1134–1156.

16. Buysse DJ, Reynolds CF III, Kupfer DJ, et al. Clinical diagnoses in 216 insomnia patients using the International Classification of Sleep Disorders (ICSD), DSM-IV, and ICD-10 categories: a report from the APA/NIMH DSM-IV field trial. Sleep. 1994; 17:630–637.

17. Gislason T and Almqvist M. Somatic disease and sleep complaints: an epidemiologic study of 3201 Swedish men. Acta Med Scand. 1987; 221:475–581.

18. Artz M and Badley TD. Treatment of sleep apnea in heart failure. Am J Respir Crit Care Med. 2006; 173(12):1300–1308.

19. Guilleminault C and Robinson A. Central sleep apnea. Neurol Clin. 1996; 14(3):611–628.

20. Badr MS, Toiber F, Skatrud JB, et al. Pharyngeal narrowing/occlusion during central sleep apnea. J Appl Physiol. 1995; 78(5):1806–1815.

21. Avidan AY. Sleep changes and disorders in the elderly patient. Curr Neurol Neurosci Rep. 2002; 2(2):178–185.

22. Hall MJ, Xie A, Rutherford R, et al. Cycle length of periodic breathing in patients with and without heart failure. Am J Respir Crit Care Med. 1996; 154:376–381.

23. Naughton MT, Benard D, Tam A, et al. The role of hyperventilation in the pathogenesis of central sleep apnea in patients with congestive heart failure. Am Rev Respir Dis. 1993; 148:330–338.

24. Weil JV. Sleep at high altitude. In: Kryger M, Roth T, and Dement WC, eds. Principles and Practice of Sleep Medicine. Philadelphia: WB Saunders. 1989; 269–275.

25. Teichtahl H, Prodromidis A, Miller B, et al. Sleep-disordered breathing in stable methadone programme patients: a pilot study. Addiction. 2001; 96:395–403.

26. Farnery R, Walker J, Cloward T, et al. Sleep-disordered breathing associated with long-term opioid therapy. Chest. 2003; 123:632–639.

27. Ancoli-Israel S and Ayalon L. Diagnosis and treatment of sleep disorders in older adults. Am J Geriatr Psychiatry. 2006; 14(2):95–103.

28. McNicholas WT and Ryan S. Obstructive sleep apnoea syndrome: translating science to clinical practice. Respirology. 2006; 11(2):136–144.

29. White DP. Sleep apnea. Proc Am Thorac Soc. 2006; 3(1):124–128.

30. The Report of an American Academy of Sleep Medicine Task Force. Sleep-related breathing disorders in adults: recommendations for syndrome definition and measurement techniques in clinical research. Sleep. 1999; 22:667–689.

31. White DP. Central sleep apnea. In: Kryger MH, Roth T, and Dement WC, eds. Principles and Practice of Sleep Medicine. 4th ed. Philadelphia: Elsevier/Saunders. 2005; 969–982.

32. Thorpy MJ. Classification of sleep disorders. In: Kryger MH, Roth T, and Dement WC, eds. Principles and Practice of Sleep Medicine. 4th ed. Philadelphia: Elsevier/Saunders. 2005; 615–625.

33. Callop N and Cassel DK. Snoring and sleep disordered breathing. In: Lee-Chiong T Jr, Sateia M, and Carskadon M, eds. Sleep Medicine. Philadelphia, PA: Hanley & Belfus. 2002; 349–355.

34. Scwab RJ, Goldberg AN, and Pack AJ. Sleep apnea syndromes. In: Fishman AP, ed. Fishman's Pulmonary Diseases and Disorders. 3rd ed. New York, NY: McGraw-Hill. 1998; 1617–1646.

35. Goldberg AN and Schwab RJ. Identifying the patient with sleep apnea: upper airway assessment and physical examination. Otolaryngol Clin North Am. 1998; 31:919–930.

36. Dyken ME and Yamada T. Narcolepsy and disorders of excessive somnolence. Prim Care. 2005; 32(2):389–413.

37. Overeem S, Mignot E, van Dijk JG, et al. Narcolepsy: clinical features, new pathophysiologic insights, and future perspectives. J Clin Neurophysiol. 2001; 18(2):78–105.

38. Arand D, Bonner M, Hurwitz T, et al. The clinical use of the MSLT and MWT. Sleep. 2005; 28(1):123–144.

39. Carskadon MA, Dement WC, Mitler MM, et al. Guidelines for the multiple sleep latency test (MSLT): a standard measure of sleepiness. Sleep. 1986; 9(4):519–524.

40. Reid KJ and Burgess HJ. Circadian rhythm sleep disorders. Prim Care. 2005; 32(2):449–473.

41. Cajochen C, Krauchi K, Wirz-Justice A, et al. Role of melatonin in the regulation of human circadian rhythms and sleep. J Neuroendocrinol. 2003; 15(4):432–437.

42. Klerman EB. Clinical aspects of human circadian rhythms. J Biol Rhythms. 2005; 20(4):375–386.

43. Waterhouse J, Reilly T, and Atkinson G. Jet-lag. Lancet. 1997; 350(9091):1611–1616.

44. Drake CL, Roehrs T, Richardson G, et al. Shift work sleep disorder: prevalence and consequences beyond that of symptomatic day workers. Sleep. 2004; 27(8):1453–1462.

45. Ohayon MM, Lemoine P, Arnaud-Briant V, et al. Prevalence and consequences of sleep disorders in a shift work population. J Psychosom Res. 2002; 53:577–583.

46. Capp PK, Pearl PL, and Lewin D. Pediatric sleep disorders. Prim Care. 2005; 32(2):549–562.

47. Malow BA. Paroxysmal events in sleep. J Clin Neurophysiol. 2002; 19(6):522–534.

48. Brooks S and Kushida CA. Behavioral phenomenas. Curr Psychiatry Rep. 2002; 4(5):363–368.

49. Mahowald MW, Bornemann MC, and Schenck CH. Parasomnias. Semin Neurol. 2004; 24(3):283–292.

50. Mahowald MW and Schenck CH. Insights from studying human sleep disorders. Nature. 2005; 437(7063):1279–1285.

51. Ohayon MM, Guilleminault C, and Priest RG. Night terrors, sleepwalking, and confusional arousals in the general population: their frequency and relationship to other sleep and mental disorders. J Clin Psychiatry. 1999; 60(4):268–277.

52. Wills L and Garcia J. Parasomnias: epidemiology and management. CNS Drugs. 2002; 16(12):803–810.

53. Nielsen TA and Zadra A. Dreaming disorders. In: Kryger MH, Roth T, and Dement WC, eds. Principles and Practice of Sleep Medicine. 3rd ed. Philadelphia: Elsevier/Saunders. 2000; 753–772.

54. Walters AS. Toward a better definition of the restless legs syndrome. The International Restless Legs Syndrome Group. Mov Disord. 1995; 10(5):634–642.

55. Michaud M, Chabli A, Lavigne G, et al. Arm restlessness in patients with restless legs syndrome. Mov Disord. 2000; 15(2):289–293.

56. Montplaisir J, Boucher S, Poirier G, et al. Clinical, polysomnographic, and genetic characteristics of restless legs syndrome: a study of 133 patients diagnosed with new standard criteria. Mov Disord. 1997; 12(1):61–65.

57. Chahine LM and Chemali ZN. Restless leg syndrome: a review. CNS Spectr. 2006; 11(7):511–520.

58. Ekbom KA. Restless leg syndrome. Neurology. 1960; 10:868–873.

59. Silber MH and Richardson JW. Multiple blood donations associated with iron deficiency in patients with restless legs syndrome. Mayo Clin Proc. 2003; 78(1):52–54.

60. Ulfberg J and Nystrom B. Restless legs syndrome in blood donors. Sleep Med. 2004; 5(2):115–118.

61. Hening W. The clinical neurophysiology of the restless legs syndrome and periodic limb movements. Part I: diagnosis, assessment, and characterization. Clin Neurophysiol. 2004; 115(9):19–65.

62. Mazza M, Della Marca G, De Risio S, et al. Sleep disorders in the elderly. Clin Ter. 2004; 155(9):391–394.

63. Coleman RM. Periodic movements in sleep (nocturnal myoclonus) and restless legs syndrome. In: Guilleminault C, ed. Sleep and Waking Disorders: Indications and Techniques. Menlo Park, CA: Addison-Wesley. 1982; 265–295.

64. Rugh J and Harlan J. Nocturnal bruxism and temporomandibular disorders. Adv Neurol. 1988; 49:329–341.

65. Rugh J. Association between bruxism and TMD. In: McNeill C, ed. Current Controversies in Temporomandibular Disorders. Chicago: Quintessence. 1992; 29.

66. Ohayon M, Li K, and Guilleminault C. Risk factors for sleep bruxism in the general population. Chest. 2001; 119:53–61.

67. Pingitore G, Chrobak V, and Petrie J. The social and pscyhologic factors of bruxism. J Prosthet Dent. 1991; 65:443–446.

68. Lobbezoo F and Naeije M. Bruxism is mainly regulated centrally, not peripherally. J Oral Rehabil. 2001; 28:1085–1089.

69. Bader G, Kampe T, and Tagdae T. Body movement during sleep in subjects with long-standing bruxing behavior. Int J Prosthodont. 2000; 13:327–333.

70. Merriam-Webster Online. Snore. Merriam-Webster Online Dictionary. 2008. Available at http://www.merriam-webster.com/dictionary/snore. Accessed September 11, 2008.

71. Young T, Peppard PE, and Gottlieb DJ. Epidemiology of obstructive sleep apnea: a population health perspective. Am J Respir Crit Care Med. 2002; 165(9):1217–1239.

72. Netzer NC, Hoegel JJ, Loube D, et al. Sleep in Primary Care International Study Group. Prevalence of symptoms and risk of sleep apnea in primary care. Chest. 2003; 124(4):1406–1414.

73. Phillipson EA and Remmers JE. American Thoracic Society Consensus Conference on indications and standards for cardiopulmonary sleep studies. Am Rev Respir Dis. 1989; 139:559–568.

74. American Sleep Disorders Association. Primary snoring. In: Hauri PJ, Task Force Chair, ed. The International Classification of Sleep Disorders, Revised: Diagnostic and Coding Manual. Rochester, MN: American Sleep Disorders Association. 1997; 195–197.

75. Hoffstein V. Snoring. In: Kryger M, Roth T, and Dement WC, eds. Principles and Practice of Sleep Medicine. Philadelphia, PA: WB Saunders. 2000; 813–826.

76. Guilleminault C, Stoohs R, Clerk A, et al. A cause of excessive daytime sleepiness: the upper-airway resistance syndrome. Chest. 1993; 104:781–787.

77. Guilleminault C, Stoohs R, and Duncan S. Snoring (I): daytime sleepiness in regular heavy snorers. Chest. 1991; 99(1):40–48.

78. Wheatley R. Definition and diagnosis of upper airway resistance syndrome. Sleep. 2000; 23(Suppl 4):S193–S196.

79. Douglas NJ. Upper airway resistance syndrome is not a distinct syndrome. Am J Respir Crit Care Med. 2000; 161(5):1413–1416.

80. Guilleminault C and Chowdhuri S. Upper airway resistance syndrome is a distinct syndrome. Am J Respir Crit Care Med. 2000; 161(5):1412–1413.

81. Gold AR, Marcus CL, Dipalo F, et al. Upper airway collapsibility during sleep in upper airway resistance syndrome. Chest. 2002; 121:1531–1540.

82. Gold AR, Dipalo F, Gold MS, et al. The symptoms and signs of upper airway resistance syndrome: a link to the functional somatic syndromes. Chest. 2003; 123:87–95.

83. Stoohs RA, Knaack L, Blum H, et al. Differences in clinical features of upper airway resistance syndrome, primary snoring, and obstructive sleep apnea/hypopnea syndrome. Sleep Med. 2008; 9:121–128.

84. Ulfberg J, Carter N, Talback M, et al. Adverse health effects among women living with heavy snorers. Health Care Women Int. 2000; 21:81–90.

85. Wolfe F, Smythe H, Yunus M, et al. The American College of Rheumatology 1990 criteria for the classification of fibromyalgia. Report of the Multicenter Criteria Committee. Arthritis Rheum. 1990; 33(2):160–172.

86. Schaefer K. Sleep disturbances and fatigue in women with fibromyalgia and chronic fatigue syndrome. J Obstet Gynecol Neonatal Nurs. 1995; 24:229–233.

87. Affleck G, Urrows S, Tennen H, et al. Sequential daily relations of sleep, pain intensity, and attention to pain among women with fibromyalgia. Pain. 1996; 68(2–3):363–368.

88. Harding H. Sleep in fibromyalgia patients: subjective and objective findings. Am J Med Sci. 1998; 315(6):367–376.

89. Moldofsky H and Lue F. The relationship of alpha and delta EEG frequencies to pain and mood in "fibrositis" patients treated with chlorpromazine and L-tryptophan. Electroencephalogr Clin Neurophysiol. 1980; 50(1–2):71–80.

90. Anch A, Lue F, MacLean A, et al. Sleep physiology and psychological aspects of fibrositis (fibromyalgia) syndrome. Can J Exp Psychol. 1991; 45:179–184.

91. Mahowald ML and Mahowald MW. Nighttime sleep and daytime functioning (sleepiness and fatigue) in less well-defined chronic rheumatic diseases with particular reference to the "alpha-delta NREM sleep anomaly". Sleep Med. 2000; 1(3):195–207.

92. Dodick D, Eross E, and Parish J. Clinical, anatomical, and physiologic relationship between sleep and headache. Headache. 2003; 43:282–292.

93. Rains J and Poceta J. Headache and sleep disorders: review and clinical implications for headache management. Headache. 2006; 46(9):1344–1361.

94. Weintraub J. Cluster headaches and sleep disorders. Curr Pain Headache Rep. 2003; 7:150–156.

95. Boardman H, Thomas E, Millson D, et al. Psychological, sleep, lifestyle and comorbid associations with headache. Headache. 2005; 45:657–669.

96. Kelman L and Rains J. Headache and sleep: examination of sleep patterns and complaints in a large clinical sample of migraineurs. Headache. 2005; 45:904–910.

97. Spierings E, Ranke A, and Honkoop P. Precipitating and aggravating factors of migraine versus tenstion-type headache. Headache. 2001; 41:554–558.

98. Houle T, Rains J, Penzien D, et al. Biobehavioral precipitants of headache: time-series analysis of stress and sleep on headache activity. Headache. 2004; 44:533–534.

99. Chervin R, Zallek S, Lin X, et al. Sleep disordered breathing in patients with cluster headache. Neurology. 2000; 54:2302–2306.

# Pediatrics and sleep-related breathing disorders

## CONCEPTUAL OVERVIEW

Sleep disorders are not exclusive to the adult population. Children and adolescents also may suffer from sleep disorders. However, sleep disorders are not as easily recognized in this group as compared to adults and therefore are frequently undiagnosed. The sleep problems are often manifested as behavioral issues, emotional concerns, or personal conflicts that are out of proportion to the actual event, such as family conflicts or stress.

The more common sleep disorders in children and adolescents involve sleep-related breathing disorders (SRBD), difficulty initiating or maintaining sleep (i.e., insomnia), periodic limb movement disorder (PLMD), or restless legs syndrome (RLS). There are other sleep disorders that may impact this age group, but the majority of them fall within these categories. SRBD is one of the major interests for the dentist.

Awareness of SRBD in the pediatric population dates back to the 1800s. A medical manuscript in 1884 indicated that mouth breathing had ill effects on children as well as adults.[1]

Another publication in 1889 noted that children presented with deafness appeared "backward and even stupid," had headaches, and would mouth breathe.[2] Also, in 1892 a medical document linked sleep and daytime performance in children with sleep-related upper airway obstruction.[3] The author stated that the "child is very stupid looking," that an "influence on mental development is striking," that the child found it "impossible to fix the attention for long at a time," and that "the expression is dull, heavy, and apathetic." Also recognized in that document were symptoms of headaches and listlessness. Others in the early half of the 1900s also found a correlation between sleep, airway obstruction, and daytime functioning. The current scientific literature is abundant with evidence that confirms these earlier anecdotal findings.

An increasing awareness in the last 20 years regarding the importance of recognizing pediatric sleep issues is demonstrated by the increase in the number of articles and textbooks that are devoted to the topic. During that period, there has been a 1,226% increase in the number of published articles related to this area.[4]

# FREQUENCY OF SLEEP DISORDERS IN THE PEDIATRIC AND ADOLESCENT POPULATION

Between 20 and 50% of the pediatric and adolescent population may have a sleep disorder.[5–8] This frequency is significant and often results in parental concern because of the clinical impact on the child's behavioral, physical, and mental health. Unfortunately, sleep disorders in this age group are not recognized and are therefore undiagnosed.

Many times the presentation of insomnia is secondary to other situations that can impact sleep, and, as such, it may actually be the presenting symptom of SRBD. The presence of insomnia, oftentimes described as individuals being poor sleepers or having insufficient sleep, may be 12–33% in this younger population.[7,9,10]

SRBD frequency in children, especially with regard to snoring or obstructive sleep apnea (OSA), has been studied the most. OSA is estimated to occur in 1–3% of children,[11] and snoring is believed to occur in 3–12% of this population, with occasional snoring being present about 20% of the time and habitual snoring being present about 10% of the time.[12]

More recently, the presence of RLS and PLMD in children has been investigated. Although the frequency is not specifically known, one study reported that about one-third of 138 adults who reported symptoms of RLS also indicated that these same symptoms were present before age 10.[13]

The key finding related to RLS in the younger age group is the association between RLS and inattentiveness, hyperactivity, and attention-deficit hyperactivity disorder (ADHD).[14]

Unlike adults, these sleep disorders may present themselves differently in this younger population. Accordingly, the sleep disorder may not be considered in conjunction with other complaints that a child may have or with signs that are evident, and thus may be overlooked. Interestingly, the utilization of health care by children with a sleep disorder is 2.6 times as compared to their matched controls.[15]

There are many health-related conditions that may be associated with a sleep disorder in a child or adolescent, but these findings may go undetected because sleep problems in this age group are oftentimes not a primary consideration (Table 4.1).

**Table 4.1**  Health-related conditions associated with sleep-related breathing disorders in children and adolescents.

| Depression | Diabetes type 2 | Allergy |
|---|---|---|
| Enuresis | Increased triglycerides | Headaches |
| Asthma | Tired/irritable ADD/ADHD | Obesity |

In addition, there are congenital conditions that indicate that a child may be at a higher risk for a sleep disorder and specifically SRBD, especially OSA (Table 4.2).

Children that present for dental care may have clinical findings that would suggest that they are at risk for SRBD.

# RECOGNITION OF SLEEP DISORDERS IN CHILDREN AND ADOLESCENTS

The recognition of a sleep disorder in children and adolescents requires the use of proper questioning techniques as well as the identification of related signs of these disorders. If a sleep disorder is suspected, then a simple questionnaire can be used to determine if the individual is at risk for a sleep disorder, but the questionnaire itself cannot be utilized as a diagnostic tool. On suspicion, a more formal referral to the child's physician or a sleep specialist is indicated.

A number of these questionnaires have been developed over the years. The Pediatric Daytime Sleepiness Scale is composed of eight questions that are most applicable to middle-school children, and it assesses the relationship between daytime sleepiness and school-related outcomes, mainly educational achievement.[16] The Pediatric Sleep-Disordered Breathing OSA-18 questionnaire evaluates quality-of-life issues related to OSA, and it looks at the symptoms as well as sleep disturbances and daytime functioning.[17] Another instrument, the Pediatric Sleep Questionnaire, has been designed as a generalized-type questionnaire that covers a wide range of issues related to sleep disruption. Table 4.3 represents a generalized pediatric sleep questionnaire.

**Table 4.2**  More common congenital conditions that predispose the child to sleep-related breathing disorders.

| Down syndrome | Pierre Robin syndrome |
|---|---|
| Prader–Willi syndrome | Achondroplasia |
| Asperger syndrome | Chiari malformation |

Source: Adapted from Sheldon SH, Ferber R, Kryger MH. Principles and Practice of Pediatric Sleep Medicine. Elsevier/Saunders. 2005; 23.

**Table 4.3**  General pediatric sleep questionnaire

Name:                    Age:          Gender:

**While Sleeping, Does Your Child:**
____ Snore more than half the time        ____ Always snore
____ Have heavy or loud breathing         ____ Snore loudly
____ Have trouble breathing or struggles to breathe
____ Ever stop breathing at night?

**Does Your Child ...?**
____ Tend to breathe through the mouth during the day
____ Have a dry mouth upon waking up in the morning
____ Occasionally wet the bed
____ Grind his/her teeth while sleeping
____ Have any bite problems or crowded teeth
____ Wake up unrefreshed in the morning
____ Have a problem with daytime sleepiness
____ Have a teacher or anyone who has commented about
      sleepiness during the day
____ Have difficulty waking up in the morning
____ Wake up with headaches
____ Have any history of growth problems
____ Have an overweight issue:   weight is____
                                 height is____
____ Complain of restless or achy legs
____ Have arms and/or legs that twitch during sleep
____ Have nightmares (more than one per week)

The Cleveland Adolescent Sleepiness Questionnaire is a more recently developed instrument and it applies to a variety of ages and sleep disorders.[18] This questionnaire may be used freely, and the authors request that the results be shared with them in an effort to refine the questionnaire over time.

A sleep disorder may need to be considered when a child presents for dental care, particularly if there are risk factors present that might indicate such a disorder.

Sleep disruption has a strong correlation to the presence of headache in both the adult and younger age group populations. One of the chief complaints that may indicate the presence of a possible sleep disorder is headache, particularly in the adolescent population.[19] For patients who had headaches, there were also complaints about sleep, which involved insufficient sleep, being sleepy during the day, having trouble falling asleep, and the presence of awakenings at night. When headaches are present, it is necessary that the clinician consider and investigate the possible existence of sleep problems as well. The most common recommendation then would be to give instructions for good sleep practices, also known as sleep hygiene.

## Sleep-related breathing disorders

SRBD consists mainly of snoring and OSA. In a child or even the adolescent patient, the presentation of snoring may appear more like heavy breathing. For an apnea or any cessation in breathing during sleep to be identified, a parent or someone else would need to observe this first hand. Therefore, the presence of apnea, like snoring, often goes undetected because most children sleep alone or in a separate room.

Another type of SRBD is termed upper airway resistance syndrome (UARS), although it is not officially recognized in the *International Classification of Sleep Disorders, Second Edition (ICSD-2)*. UARS may appear to be OSA; however, the key differences are that the respiratory events of UARS are related to an arousal and there are no distinct apneas or hypopneas.[20] In addition, the level of blood oxygen, also known as oxygen saturation, does not decrease with UARS.

The recognition of SRBD in a child can also be related to simply mouth breathing alone.[21] This type of breathing pattern during sleep appears to have an almost identical affect on the quality of sleep, and thus may result in very similar symptoms as a definitive SRBD.

The presentation of symptoms or signs associated with SRBD in children can be recognized on the basis of either the daytime or nighttime findings (Table 4.4).

One study outlined the presentation of symptoms associated with SRBD that were divided into three age groups: preschool, preadolescent, and adolescent (Table 4.5).[22]

Because SRBD has not been a typical or usual consideration when evaluating pediatric patients, the American Academy of Pediatrics (AAP)

**Table 4.4** Symptoms and findings at nighttime and daytime in children with sleep-related breathing disorders.

| Nighttime | Daytime |
|---|---|
| Snoring | Neurocognitive impairment |
| Bruxism | ADHD and ADD |
| Awakenings | Hyperactivity |
| Mouth breathing | Behavioral issues (irritable) |
| Nightmares | Tired/poor school performance |

**Table 4.5** Clinical manifestations of sleep-related breathing disorders in three age groups—up to the age of 18; based on the review of 189 charts.

| Associated problem | Preschool (n = 41) | Preadolescent (n = 91) | Adolescent (n = 51) |
|---|---|---|---|
| Daytime fatigue | 30% | 50% | 71.1% |
| Excessive daytime sleepiness (EDS) | 38.7% | 59.2% | 80.4% |
| Sleep-onset insomnia | 40% | 21% | 48.1% |
| Nocturnal sleep disruption | 85.3% | 69.5% | 70.6% |
| Nightmare | 12.5% | 19.7% | 21.3% |
| Sleep walking | 9.4% | 24% | 12.8% |
| Enuresis | 40.7% | 31.9% | 20.5% |
| Sleep bruxism | 50% | 49.3% | 23.9% |
| ADHD | 13.8% | 29.4% | 40.9% |
| Morning headaches | 9.7% | 12% | 19.1% |
| Delayed sleep phase syndrome | 0% | 4.1% | 30.6% |
| Mean AHI | 16.4 (±16.8) | 10.3 (±13.3) | 16.2 (±22.9) |
| Mean RDI | 16.6 (±15.7) | 11.1 (±12.2) | 16.3 (±21.8) |

Source: Adapted from Kim J, Won C, Guilleminault C. The clinical manifestation of sleep-disordered breathing in children and adolescent. Sleep. 2007; 30(Abstract Supplement):86.

developed a guideline for the diagnosis and management of SRBD in this age group of patients.[23] The guidelines recommend that

- all children be screened for snoring;
- in the presence of a cardiorespiratory health condition, the child should have a more extensive evaluation;
- diagnostic evaluation be conducted to determine if the risk for OSA is present, most often resulting in an overnight sleep study.

This type of guideline can easily be implemented in the dental setting by anyone who treats pediatric patients.

Treatment for OSA in children is most often a tonsillectomy and adenoidectomy when those anatomical structures are enlarged because of their potential to be interfering with the airway. This is the first line of treatment and often the most successful. Following this surgical intervention, in many instances the symptoms are reversed and no further treatment is indicated.

## CLINICAL FINDINGS

Clinically, at the time of an oral evaluation, there are some signs that a patient may be at risk for a sleep disorder and specifically SRBD. Prior to the clinical evaluation, the history is a critical component in the recognition process.

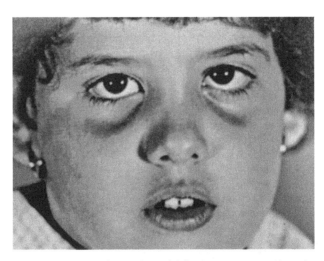

**Figure 4.1**   An example of an adenoidal face. (Meyer B and Marks MD. Stigmata of Respiratory Tract Allergies. Kalamazoo, MI: Upjohn Co. 1977. Used with permission from Pfizer Inc.)

There are facial features that indicate a risk for SRBD. The most common of these are the following:

- *Adenoidal faces:* This is a condition where the face is rounded with an often blank stare (Figure 4.1).
- *Allergic shiners:* These are the dark circles that are often found under the eyes. They are related to a reduction or absence in nasal breathing with an increased amount of mouth breathing (Figure 4.2).

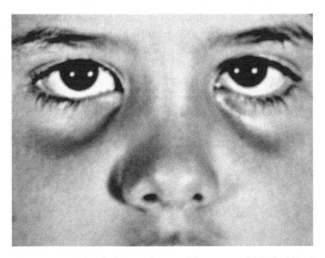

**Figure 4.2**   An example of allergic shiners. (Meyer B and Marks MD. Stigmata of Respiratory Tract Allergies. Kalamazoo, MI: Upjohn Co. 1977. Used with permission from Pfizer Inc.)

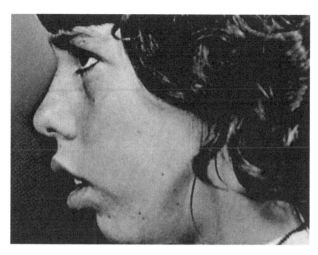

**Figure 4.3**   An example of poor or inadequate (open) lip seal. (Meyer B and Marks MD. Stigmata of Respiratory Tract Allergies. Kalamazoo, MI: Upjohn Co. 1977. Used with permission from Pfizer Inc.)

- *Poor or inadequate lip seal:* In this situation, the lips are found to be apart with the appearance of difficulty in the ability to maintain a lip seal (Figure 4.3).
- *Small nares:* The opening to the nasal airway is small and appears constricted (Figure 4.4).
- *Nasal crease:* This is a horizontal line that goes across the nose above the tip of the nose. Oftentimes this may be associated with the allergic salute, which is a gesture associated with a repetitive action of wiping the nose due to the feeling of a constant drainage. This clinical feature may be associated with an allergy (Figure 4.5).

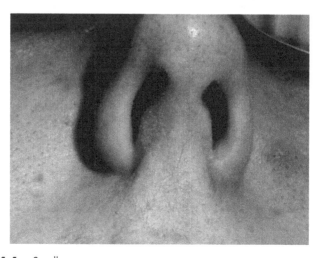

**Figure 4.4**   Small nares.

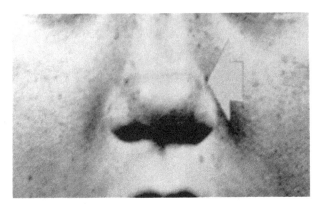

**Figure 4.5**    An example of nasal crease; note the arrow pointing to the line across the nose. (Meyer B and Marks MD. Stigmata of Respiratory Tract Allergies. Kalamazoo, MI: Upjohn Co. 1977. Used with permission from Pfizer Inc.)

On clinical evaluation of the intraoral structures, there are a number of findings that indicate the increased potential for being at risk for SRBD. The ones most commonly encountered are the following:

- Bruxism or worn teeth (Figure 4.6)
- Crossbite and/or high palate (Figure 4.7)
- Scalloped tongue (Figure 4.8)
- Swollen or enlarged uvula (Figure 4.9)
- Enlarged tonsils (Figure 4.10)
- Deep or collapsed bite (Figure 4.11)

Neck size may also be a factor, but this has not been as clearly defined as it has for adults.

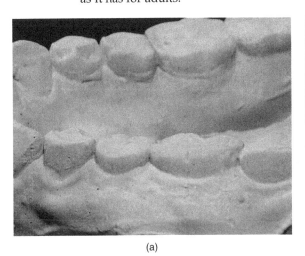

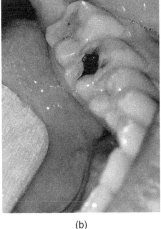

(a)                                                        (b)

**Figure 4.6**    Worn posterior teeth due to severe bruxism over many years as seen (a) on a study model and (b) clinically on the molars.

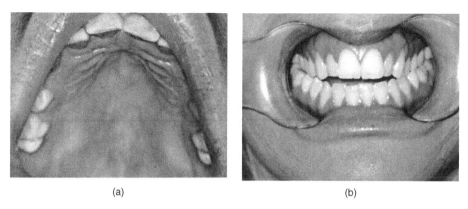

(a)                                                    (b)

**Figure 4.7** High palatal vault often accompanied by a posterior crossbite:
(a) high or deep palate and (b) posterior crossbite oftentimes seen with a high palate.

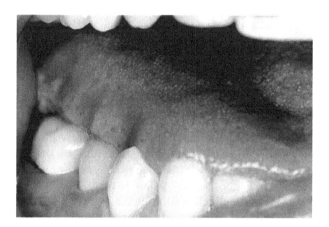

**Figure 4.8** Scalloping (crenations) along the lateral border of the tongue.

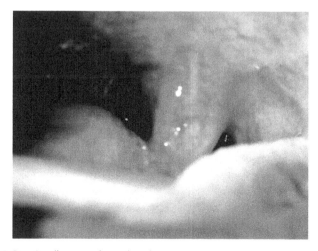

**Figure 4.9** Swollen or enlarged uvula.

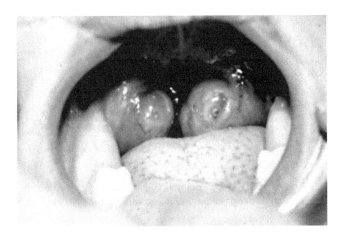

**Figure 4.10**    Swollen or enlarged tonsils.

## SLEEP STUDIES FOR CHILDREN

Sleep studies for children are the most effective means by which a determination of OSA can be made. In this age group, the data values that relate to the adult population do not apply here. Although a standardized set of values do not exist, there are guidelines by the American Thoracic Society (ATS) regarding what degree of apnea or hyponea should be present to make a diagnosis of OSA (Table 4.6).[24]

The ATS guidelines outline the severity of sleep apnea by apnea index, and they also report that an apnea–hypopnea index (AHI) greater than 5

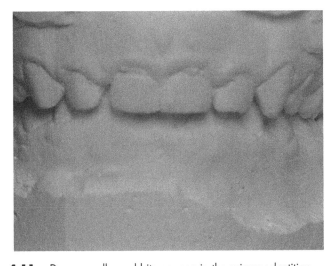

**Figure 4.11**    Deep or collapsed bite as seen in the primary dentition.

**Table 4.6** Polysomnographic (sleep study) values for sleep apnea in the pediatric population.

| Diagnosis | Apnea index (AI) events per hour | Oxygen saturation |
|---|---|---|
| Mild | 1–4 | 86–91% |
| Moderate | 5–10 | 76–85% |
| Severe | >10 | ≤75% |

*Source:* Adapted from American Thoracic Society. Standards and indications for cardiopulmonary sleep studies in children. Am J Respir Crit Care Med. 1996; 153:866–878.

with a drop in the blood oxygen level below 92% also indicates that OSA is present. The most likely reason for these values to be lower than those for the adult population is that OSA is a progressive disease, and the symptoms that affect the child can worsen over time if they are not addressed.

# CONSEQUENCES OF SLEEP DISRUPTION

Sleep disruption does not need to imply that the sleep is disrupted at some period between initiating sleep and waking up. It can also be related to an inadequate number of hours of sleep, and a reduction in total sleep time has the potential to lead to a variety of health-related consequences. One study found that among children that were 9–12 years of age who did not get 9 hours of sleep a night, the incidence for the onset of obesity was increased.[25] In a study of children who were 7 years of age, if they slept less than 9 hours per night, they were three times more likely to be overweight or obese when compared to similar children who slept more than 9 hours.[26]

The reverse is also true. Children who are obese or overweight tend to be at a higher risk for SRBD, particularly OSA. However, sleep issues associated with obesity may be overlooked, and the focus may turn to diet and exercise in lieu of the number of hours of sleep or if snoring is present.

A recent study resulted in an AAP policy statement regarding obese children and the need to screen for elevated lipid levels.[27] Outlined in the study was the associated risk that exists for diabetes type 2, cardiovascular disease, and hypertension. In addition, the policy statement emphasized the need for dietary considerations as well as the need for exercise.

Growth can be impacted by poor sleep quality, especially by the reduction or absence in nonrapid eye movement sleep and particularly deep sleep or delta sleep, also known as restorative sleep.[28] This impaired sleep quality may lead to a decreased level of growth hormone that can be associated with SRBD, and it can also be attributed to an increase in the size of the tonsils and adenoids. The compromised airway from the enlarged tonsils and adenoids may lead to sleep disruption directly associated with breathing disorders during sleep.

In addition, the enlarged tonsils can impact the ability of the child to eat and swallow and thus result in a decreased appetite. It is often found that children with airway problems are deficient in their growth as compared to their matched controls. One study found that growth failure was at least twice the expected norm in children who presented for surgical removal of the tonsils and adenoids or who had sleep symptoms.[29]

When children, and particularly adolescents, have difficulty initiating sleep, also known as sleep onset insomnia, the potential for having an increased risk for sleep disruption and related symptoms increases. Most of the time, this situation is associated with a sleep disorder common to adolescents known as delayed sleep phase syndrome,[30] which is a condition classified as a circadian rhythm disorder. In this situation, the individual attempts to go to bed and to sleep at a set specific time; however, because of a natural alteration in their internal clock, they are not truly ready to initiate sleep. The subsequent outcome is that they lie awake in bed despite the attempts to fall asleep. Consequently, they fall asleep a few hours later than was desired, which can cause difficulty in waking up at a set time the next morning. This may result in mood swings, irritability, symptoms similar to attention deficit disorder (ADD) and attention-deficit hyperactivity disorder (ADHD), depression, daytime hypersomnolence or excessive daytime sleepiness (EDS), and, where applicable, an increased risk for a motor vehicle accident.

Sleep disruption and the lack of sufficient sleep may also lead to inattention that can result in problems with learning and cognition.[31] This may be observed as behavioral or poor school performance, and it may result in an increased risk for accidents or injury.

# OTHER SLEEP DISORDERS OF INTEREST

## Insomnia

Insomnia is classically defined as the inability to initiate sleep or maintain sleep. Symptoms or signs that a child may be at risk for insomnia include depression, anxiety, mood changes, painful conditions, and headaches. Insomnia may actually be diagnosed as one of these other medical conditions as opposed to the actual sleep disorder that is involved. Oftentimes these conditions are recognized as a consequence of medication(s) that has been prescribed as opposed to the actual condition for which the medication is indicated. In addition, there may be times when insomnia is thought to be simply a "normal" consequence of the individual's age, especially in the teenage years.

If a child or adolescent has difficulty with their sleep and this appears to be related to insomnia, then attention should be directed toward the sleep

**Table 4.7**  Recommended hours of sleep for children and adolescents.

| Age range | Ideal hours of sleep |
|---|---|
| Infants | |
| 0–3 months | 15–17 |
| 3–18 months | 13–15 |
| Toddlers | |
| 1–3 years | 12–14 |
| 3–5 years | 11–13 |
| 5–12 years | 10–11 |
| Adolescents (early teens) | 8.5–9.25 |
| Teens (mainly high school) | 8.5–9.5 |

*Source:* Adapted from National Sleep Foundation. Available at www.nsf.org. 2009.

disorder. When a child simply gets a reduced number of hours of sleep, then his or her general health can suffer. The lack of adequate sleep in terms of the number of hours for children and adolescents needs to be addressed by the parents. However, for the parents to facilitate this, they must know what the proper number of hours of sleep should be for the appropriate age group. Studies have looked at this situation, and, in general, the number of hours of sleep varies with age, and it is believed to be more than that required for an adult (Table 4.7).

A National Sleep Foundation's research report demonstrated that adolescents clearly do not get an adequate number of hours of sleep as recommended.[32] Only 20% of teenagers get the necessary 9 hours of sleep, and they get fewer and fewer hours as they progress from sixth grade to the senior year in high school. In addition, parents are not aware of the number of hours of sleep that teenagers are actually getting. In a study from the 2006 Sleep in America poll, parents felt that adolescents were getting adequate sleep 90% of the time while 44% of those same adolescents felt that they were getting adequate sleep.[33]

## Restless legs syndrome and periodic limb movement disorder

The presentation of RLS and PLMD need to be evaluated or considered. The best way to determine if this is present is by history and by recognition of clinical findings that may be present. Oftentimes the recognition of the risk for RLS and PLMD is based on the possible outcome as opposed to the specific symptoms.

RLS is most often present later in the day or at the time when the individual first attempts to initiate sleep. The most commonly occurring symptoms are the inability to sit or lay still, frequent movement of the legs, and a feeling of an achy or crawling sensation in the legs.[34] Many times the presentation of these symptoms is passed off as leg pain or may be referred to as growing pains.

In conjunction with RLS, patients may have SRBD. The symptoms from the breathing disorder are the first ones to be recognized and may include the feeling of being tired, inattentiveness or ADD/ADHD-type symptoms, irritability or mood swings, and even poor school performance. The initiating factor in the presentation of these symptoms is the sleep disruption that leads to arousals during sleep. This fragmented sleep pattern results in a reduction of the quality of sleep and hence the symptoms begin to appear.

Clinically, it is possible that the presentation of evidence that suggests a tooth grinding or bruxism habit may also be related. Sleep bruxism and its relationship to RLS in adults may be present in 9–11% of the adult population.[35] Even though this has not been well defined in the pediatric population, the general relationship may apply.

PLMD most often occurs during sleep, and it is a condition where the legs and possibly the arms move or jerk involuntarily during sleep. The recognition of this is most often dependent on a bed partner. It is possible that the individual themselves might feel that their sleep is restless, thus indicating its presence.

Both RLS and PLMD originate in the central nervous system and are associated with the dopamine centers in the brain. Because of their close association with sleep bruxism, the occurrence of these two conditions may also be precipitated by some foods, beverages, or medications. Most commonly recognized are cigarettes, caffeine, amphetamines, and mainly selective serotonin reuptake inhibitor antidepressants. In addition, a lowered ferritin level is a possibility as a precipitating factor.

## Narcolepsy

Narcolepsy presents as brief attacks of uncontrollable sleepiness or EDS. Oftentimes this sleep disorder may go unrecognized and may even be thought to be symptoms associated with SRBD. The age of onset is typically between 15 and 30 years, and the disorder may not be diagnosed until the third or fourth decade of life. There may be a family history of others with it as well.

The presence of narcolepsy is 3–16 per 10,000, and it usually presents in the second decade of life.[36] One of the classic symptoms is cataplexy, also known as a sudden muscle weakness, particularly of the legs and trunk, and it occurs in association with some emotional stimulus such as laughter, fear, or rage.

Many times pharmaceutical stimulants similar to those used for managing ADD or ADHD can be used to treat the narcolepsy. In addition, there are other more specific medications that can be used to treat this particular sleep disorder and they should be prescribed by a physician, such as a sleep specialist, who is well-versed in their use and who will provide adequate follow-up care.

# TREATMENT STRATEGIES

The treatment of pediatric sleep disorders, especially with the management of an SRBD, is frequently a multidisciplinary approach involving the pediatrician or family physician, an otolaryngologist, the general dentist, a pediatric dentist, an orthodontist, and at times a speech therapist. Complete evaluation and diagnosis of sleep disorders need to be referred to the appropriate medical specialist, and oftentimes the role of the dentist is relegated to the recognition and initial education of the parents and the patient.

The actual treatment often may not take place as early in the developmental process as it should because of the lack of initial identification of the problem along with the need for one of the practitioners to coordinate the care that is needed. In every case, the first step in this process is the recognition of a sleep disorder, especially SRBD. Any dentist who sees children is well-positioned to recognize a developing situation and propose the necessary treatment.

## First step is recognition

The recognition of a SRBD involves the detection of a variety of signs that the possible disorder exists. Many times these are subtle in nature, but, more often than not, they involve the growth and development of the child. The potential for early recognition of SRBD and the appropriate treatment of the upper airway, once there is a recognized problem, may be a means of preventing the development of OSA as an adult.[21]

Because SRBD is the condition with which the dentist will be involved, the recognition of related symptoms as well as clinical findings is essential. In addition, various pediatric questionnaires should be utilized whenever necessary along with an ongoing review of the patient's health history.

Subsequently, the development of a treatment plan as well as making the necessary referrals are in order.

## Treatment options

The treatment specifically as it relates to SRBD should be initiated as soon as a problem is recognized, which typically involves a number of other health care providers that include a variety of medical specialties.

### Tonsillectomy and adenoidectomy

The surgical removal of the tonsils and adenoids has and continues to be the first line of treatment. This intervention has been recognized as the primary treatment for children who snore and may be at risk for OSA.[23,37] One study found that the success rate for this procedure, as measured by sleep study results, demonstrated that the AHI was improved by

95% and that the normalization of the sleep study occurred 82.9% of the time.[38]

The removal of the tonsils and adenoids also has an impact on other factors related to SRBD. It has been shown that behavioral problems associated with SRBD were improved after this procedure.[39] Another study demonstrated that behavioral issues such as hyperactivity, ADHD, and EDS were improved 1 year after the surgery was performed.[40] It is interesting to note that children with ADHD were three times as likely to snore, a common finding associated with enlarged tonsils and adenoids, when compared to non-ADHD children.[41]

Snoring by itself should not be overlooked. Even though behavioral symptoms may not be present, the recognition of snoring has been found to be a strong risk factor for the presentation of hyperactivity over a 4-year period.[42] This finding is significant since the recognition of ADHD has increased significantly between 1970 and 2000 during which time the reported prevalence has gone from 1.7% to a range of 5–10%.[43]

The indications for tonsillectomy and adenoidectomy have been documented.[44] These include hyperplasia of these structures, OSA, failure to thrive, and abnormal growth of the craniofacial structures. Additional considerations identified include suspicion of other pathology, dysphagia, speech changes, and perhaps even halitosis.

## Dental and orthodontic treatment

Dental and orthodontic treatment is intended to enhance growth and development as well as to improve the airway. There may be instances, though, when this will only prove beneficial after the tonsils and adenoids have been removed.

One of the primary means by which the airway may be improved is with palatal expansion. Studies have demonstrated that palatal expansion improved snoring and daytime hypersomnolence or EDS.[45,46] Another study looked at children who had a mean AHI of 12.2. After 4 months, all the children had an AHI that was less than 1.0 and had an improvement in their nasal airway. The mean cross-section expansion was 4.32 mm and a variation of less than 1 mm. A more current investigation looked at adenoidectomy and palatal expansion in combination.[47] These two procedures were found to be mutually beneficial in the resolution of the symptoms as well as the OSA. Also of importance in this study is the recognition of the team treatment from various disciplines. The article also points out the need for an orthodontic treatment plan to focus on the airway and not just the dental and occlusal conditions. If the patient has an already existing compromised airway, then the use of techniques such as extraction and headgear should be avoided because of their impact on anteroposterior development. Instead, orthodontics should be considered as a treatment directed toward improvement of the airway on a long-term basis. Furthermore, it is indicated that when a pediatric patient has OSA or is at risk, then a facial analysis may be warranted.

In order for an awareness of the significance of airway compromise to be recognized, questions related to the airway must be performed on a regular basis. One study reviewed the impact of snoring and sleep disturbance in the orthodontic setting.[48] It found that 17% of the patients were habitual snorers, and the patients who were mouth breathers were three times as likely to snore. In addition, if they slept with their heads tipped back, they were more likely to have headaches and were more likely to have frequent colds and cough.

### Other considerations

In addition to the aforementioned treatment considerations, it may be necessary to involve other health care providers. These other providers may include speech therapy and more importantly myofunctional tongue therapy to address the tongue posture, tongue thrusting, any speech-related issues, and the swallowing pattern. Physical therapy may also be necessary to address postural considerations as well as cervical dysfunction. In both these situations, the patient would benefit the most from a home exercise program that is designed to reinforce and maintain the intended outcomes of these therapies.

Another association that should be considered is the nasal airway and allergy. It is important for the patient to be able to adequately breathe through the nose, especially during sleep, because of the affects that allergy may have on the nasal structures. Lack of adequate nasal breathing leads to habitual mouth breathing, and this may progress to snoring and OSA. Addressing the nasal airway has been shown to improve the sleep in patients with OSA.[49] If the nasal airway is compromised, then allergy, structural conditions, and even asthma and reflux need to be considered. This would best be done by a referral to an allergist, otolaryngologist, or the primary care physician.

## CONCLUSION

Sleep disorders and particularly SRBD are not uncommon to the pediatric population. Many times the presentation of the patient is with symptoms that do not directly indicate that a sleep disorder may be present, and subsequently the sleep disorder is unrecognized. Because dentists are involved with the head, neck, and oral cavity, there may be signs that a patient is at risk, but the subtle signs or symptoms go undetected.

The dentist who treats children needs to include a clinical examination and questioning for signs or symptoms that may indicate a sleep disorder and thus make the necessary referral to the physician. This can only be of benefit to the child in the long run and it may improve their quality of life.

The dentist who is involved with any type of treatment that involves the airway or growth and development, particularly orthodontics, needs to be especially vigilant of the airway and the implications of the proposed treatment on the airway. The possibility of preventing the development of OSA as the child reaches adulthood is intriguing.

# REFERENCES

1. Wagner C. Habitual-Mouth Breathing: Its Causes, Effects, and Treatment. 2nd ed. Albany, N.Y.: Werner The Voice Press. 1884.
2. Hill M. On some causes of backwardness and stupidity in children. Brit Med J. 1889; 2:711–712.
3. Osler W. Chronic tonsillitis. In: Osler W, ed. The Principles and Practice of Medicine. New York: D. Appleton and Company. 1892; 335–339.
4. Marcus C. And miles to go before we sleep. Sleep Med Rev. 2006; 10(2):79–81.
5. Sheldon SH, Ferber R, and Kryger MH. Epidemiology of sleep disorders during childhood. In: Kryger MH, Roth T, and Dement WC, eds. Principles and Practice of Pediatric Sleep Medicine. Philadelphia: Elsevier/Saunders. 2005; 29.
6. Owens JA and Mindell JA. Sleep in the pediatric practice. In: Owens JA and Mindell JA, eds. A Clinical Guide to Pediatric Sleep. Philadelphia: Lippincott Williams & Wilkins. 2003; 2.
7. Anders TF, Halpern LF, and Hua J. Sleeping through the night: a developmental perspective. Pediatrics. 1992; 90:554–560.
8. Beltramini AU and Hertzig ME. Sleep and bedtime behavior in preschool-aged children. Pediatrics. 1983; 71:153–158.
9. Owens JA and Mindell JA. Insomnia. In: Owens JA and Mindell JA, eds. A Clinical Guide to Pediatric Sleep. Philadelphia: Lippincott Williams & Wilkins. 2003; 157.
10. Hoban TF. Sleep and its disorders in children. Semin Neurol. 2004; 24:327–340.
11. Redline S, Tishler PV, Schluchter M, et al. Risk factors for sleep-disordered breathing in children: association with obesity, race, and respiratory problems. Am J Respir Crit Care Med. 1999; 159:1527–1532.
12. Owens JA and Mindell JA. Obstructive sleep apnea and sleep disordered breathing. In: Owens JA and Mindell JA, eds. A Clinical Guide to Pediatric Sleep. Philadelphia: Lippincott Williams & Wilkins. 2003; 108.
13. Walters AS, Hickey K, Maltzman J, et al. A questionnaire study of 138 patients with restless legs syndrome: the "Night-Walkers" survey. Neurology. 1996; 46:92–95.
14. Chervin RD, Archbold KH, Dillon JE, et al. Associations between symptoms of inattention, hyperactivity, restless legs, and periodic leg movements. Sleep. 2002; 25(5): 213–218.

15. Halbower AC and Mahone EM. Neuropsychological morbidity linked to childhood sleep-disordered breathing. Sleep Med Rev. 2006; 10:97–107.

16. Drake C, Nickel C, Burduvali E, et al. The Pediatric Daytime Sleepiness Scale (PDSS): sleep habits and school outcomes in middle-school children. Sleep. 2003; 26(4):455–458.

17. Franco RA, Rosenfeld RM, and Rao M. Quality of life for children with obstructive sleep apnea. Otolaryngol Head Neck Surg. 2000; 123:9–16.

18. Spilsbury JC, Drotar D, Rosen C, et al. The cleveland adolescent sleepiness questionnaire: a new measure to assess excessive daytime sleepiness in adolescents. J Clin Sleep Med. 2007; 3(6):603–612.

19. Luc ME, Birnberg JM, Reddick D, et al. Characterization of symptoms of sleep disorders in children with headache. Pediatr Neurol. 2006; 34(1):7–12.

20. Guilleminault C, Stoohs R, Clerk A, et al. A cause of excessive daytime sleepiness: the upper airway resistance syndrome. Chest. 1993; 104:781–787.

21. Guilleminault C, Li K, Quo S, et al. A prospective study on the surgical outcomes of children with sleep-disordered breathing. Sleep. 2004; 27(1):95–100.

22. Kim J, Won C, and Guilleminault C. The clinical manifestation of sleep-disordered breathing in children and adolescent. Sleep. 2007; 30(Abstract Supplement):86.

23. American Academy of Pediatrics. Clinical practice guideline: diagnosis and management of childhood obstructive sleep apnea syndrome. Pediatrics. 2002; 109:712–724.

24. American Thoracic Society. Standards and indications for cardiopulmonary sleep studies in children. Am J Respir Crit Care Med. 1996; 153:866–878.

25. Lumeng JC, Somashekar D, Appugliese D, et al. Shorter sleep duration is associated with increased risk for being overweight at ages 9 to 12 years. Pediatrics. 2007; 120(5):1020–1029.

26. Nixon GM, Thompson JMD, Han DY, et al. Short sleep duration in middle childhood: risk factors and consequences. Sleep. 2008; 31(1):71–78.

27. Daniels SR, Greer FR, and the Committee on Nutrition. Lipid screening and cardiovascular health in childhood. Pediatrics. 2008; 122(1):198–208.

28. Ahlqvist-Rastad J, Hutcrantz E, and Melander H. Body growth in relation to tonsillar enlargement and tonsillectomy. Int J Otorhinolaryngol. 1992; 24:55–61.

29. Bonuck K, Parikh S, and Bassila M. Growth failure and sleep disordered breathing: a review of the literature. Int J Pediatr Otorhinolaryngol. 2006; 70(5):769–778.

30. American Academy of Sleep Medicine. The International Classification of Sleep Disorders, Second Edition. Westchester, IL: American Academy of Sleep Medicine. 2005; 118–120.

31. Ebert CS and Drake AF. The impact of sleep-disordered breathing on cognition and behavior in children: a review and meta-synthesis of the literature. Otolaryngol Head Neck Surg. 2004; 131:814–826.

32. National Sleep Foundation. Adolescent Sleep Needs and Patterns, Research Report and Resource Guide. Washington, DC: National Sleep Foundation. 2000; 1–30.

33. National Sleep Foundation. Sleep in America Poll. Washington, DC: National Sleep Foundation. 2006; 1–77.

34. Konofal E, Corteses S, Marchand M, et al. Impact of restless legs syndrome and iron deficiency on attention deficit/hyperactivity disorder in children. Sleep Med. 2007; 8(7–8):711–715.

35. Lavigne GJ and Montplaisir JY. Restless legs syndrome and sleep bruxism: prevalence and association among canadians. Sleep. 1994; 17(8):739–743.

36. Owens JA and Mindell JA. Narcolepsy. In: Owens JA and Mindell JA, eds. A Clinical Guide to Pediatric Sleep. Philadelphia: Lippincott Williams & Wilkins. 2003; 135.

37. Potsic WP, Pasquariello PS, Baranak CC, et al. Relief of upper airway obstruction by adenotonsillectomy. Otolaryngol Head Neck Surg. 1986; 94:476–480.

38. Brietzke SE and Gallagher D. The effectiveness of tonsillectomy and adenoidectomy in the treatment of pediatric obstructive sleep apnea/hypopnea syndrome: a meta-analysis. Otolaryngol Head Neck Surg. 2006; 134(6):979–984.

39. Mitchell RB and Kelly J. Behavioral changes in children with mild sleep-disordered breathing of obstructive sleep apnea after adenotonsillectomy. Laryngoscope. 2007; 117(9):1685–1688.

40. Chervin RD, Ruzicka DL, Giordani BJ, et al. Sleep-disordered breathing, behavior, and cognition in children before and after adenotonsillectomy. Pediatrics. 2006; 117(4):e769–e778.

41. Sheldon SH, Ferber R, and Kryger MH. Attention deficit, hyperactivity, and sleep disorders. In: Kryger MH, Roth T, and Dement WC, eds. Principles and Practice of Pediatric Sleep Medicine. Philadelphia: Elsevier/Saunders. 2005; 163.

42. Chervin RD, Ruzicka DL, Archbold KH, et al. Snoring predicts hyperactivity four years later. Sleep. 2005; 28(7):885–890.

43. Lewin DS and Di Pinto M. Sleep disorders and ADHD: shared and common phenotypes. Sleep. 2004; 27(2):188–189.

44. Darrow DH and Siemens C. Indications for tonsillectomy and adenoidectomy. Laryngoscope. 2002; 112(8 Pt 2):6–10.

45. Cistulli PA, Palmisano RG, and Poole MD. Treatment of obstructive sleep apnea syndrome by rapid maxillary expansion. Sleep. 1998; 21(8):831–835.

46. Pirelli P, Saponara M, and Guilleminault C. Rapid maxillary expansion in children with obstructive sleep apnea syndrome. Sleep. 2004; 27(4):761–766.

47. Guilleminault C, Quo S, Huynh NT, et al. Orthodontic expansion treatment and adenotonsillectomy in the treatment of obstructive sleep apnea in pre-pubertal children. Sleep. 31(7):953–957.

48. Nelson S and Kulnis R. Snoring and sleep disturbance among children from an orthodontic setting. Sleep Breath. 2001; 5(2):63–70.

49. Friedman M, Tanyeri H, Lim JW, et al. Effect of improved nasal breathing on obstructive sleep apnea. Otolaryngol Head Neck Surg. 2000; 122(1):71–74.

# 5

# Medical and dental conditions related to sleep-related breathing disorders

## CONCEPTUAL OVERVIEW

Research during the past decade has confirmed that sleep disorders adversely affect various physiological systems, including cardiovascular, metabolic, psychobiologic, endocrine, nervous, and immune.

Almost from the onset of the recognition of sleep-related breathing disorders (SRBD) in patients, there has been an awareness that this particular sleep disorder could increase the risk for health-related consequences. Although cardiovascular disease has been found to be one of the more significant consequences of SRBD, the risk for other health problems has also been demonstrated.

The most widely recognized and often referred to study regarding the health-related risks with SRBD is the Sleep Heart Health Study.[1] Additional studies have also been published that support the association between SRBD and the risk for many common medical conditions.

## HEALTH CONSEQUENCES ASSOCIATED WITH SRBD

An increasing prevalence of metabolic syndrome is linked with SRBD. Metabolic syndrome is the term for a group of risk factors that are associated with specific health issues, including but not limited to cardiovascular disease, diabetes, and stroke. This syndrome, which is also known as Syndrome X, insulin resistance, and obesity syndrome, may be associated with SRBD. In one study, the presence of metabolic syndrome was found to be almost 40% greater in SRBD subjects than in control subjects.[2] There is ongoing research and discussion in the medical field relative to further clarifying this syndrome.

The criterion by which metabolic syndrome is diagnosed is predicated on an individual having a minimum of three of the five following metabolic risk factors:[3] (1) increased girth of the waist or having a gut with an increased body mass index (BMI), (2) increased blood levels of triglycerides, (3) decreased blood levels of high-density lipoprotein (HDL) cholesterol, (4) increased blood pressure, and (5) impaired fasting glucose.

The prevalence of diabetes and obesity in the United States is increasing, and the link of these risk factors to metabolic syndrome lends to the estimation of almost 50 million adults with this syndrome.[4] In addition, obesity is associated with other health problems such as increased insulin resistance, increased levels of cholesterol and triglycerides, and a variety of other health consequences, primarily related to cardiovascular disease.

The most widely acknowledged association with SRBD and even just sleep loss or restriction relates to the presence of obesity,[5–7] although SRBD does not have to be present for obesity to occur. Sleep restriction or a decrease in adequate hours of sleep may also lead to the obesity.[8,9] The sleep loss and obesity association is not exclusive to adults. Obesity in children and adolescents is an increasing concern and appears to also be related to a lack of adequate number of hours of sleep.[10,11]

Not all patients with SRBD are obese. Even the nonobese are at risk for similar health problems, mostly associated with short sleep duration.[12] An increase in abdominal girth or central (visceral) size is the one common finding that most often indicates SRBD as increasing the risk for health-related consequences.[9]

## Hypertension

Since the early 1990s, studies have recognized that an individual with SRBD is at an increased risk for elevated blood pressure or hypertension. One study looked at the incidence of hypertension in obstructive sleep apnea (OSA) patients independent of obesity,[13] and it demonstrated the following: (1) the incidence of elevated blood pressure existed in 20–70% of OSA patients, (2) significant OSA was found in 30–40% of hypertensive patients, and (3) nocturnal SRBD was more closely related to elevated blood pressure.

Arousals from sleep are also a factor in the elevation of blood pressure.[14] These repeated arousals are associated with an increase in blood pressure during the day, and they appear to be related to an increase in sympathetic activity or tone that occurred during sleep and resulted in a rise in daytime blood pressure.[15] The Sleep Heart Health Study further confirmed an association between SRBD and hypertension.[1]

Snoring alone can also lead to an elevation in blood pressure. A study demonstrated that snoring without any significant apnea or hypopnea can result in hypertension, but the risk is lower.[16] Another study showed that SRBD and the risk for hypertension were greater in younger males than in males over the age of 60.[17] Given the fact that snoring over time may lead to OSA, this should not be taken lightly.

## Cardiovascular disease

The development of cardiovascular disease takes on a variety of related conditions, all of which have been found to be prevalent in the presence of SRBD. Studies may vary on the degree of risk, but it is generally agreed upon that SRBD is a significant factor in the presentation of cardiovascular disease.

### Arrhythmias

Various arrhythmias have been documented during episodes of OSA, and they are resolved with continuous positive airway pressure therapy.[18] In addition, bradycardia and tachycardia have been implicated as associated with OSA. Hypoxia's main outcome is bradycardia. Arrhythmia appears to be associated with oxygen desaturation, is common in patients with coronary heart disease, and appears to resolve with the management of the apnea.

### Atrial fibrillation

There is an association between sleep apnea and the presence of atrial fibrillation.[19] The odds ratio for the association of atrial fibrillation with OSA was found to be 2.19. All the patients studied were similar, especially as it related to the presence of diabetes, hypertension, and congestive heart failure (CHF).

### Atherosclerosis, endothelial dysfunction, and coronary heart disease

OSA and the presence of coronary artery disease is significant. A study found that in a population of patients who had symptomatic angina diagnosed with angiography, 30.5% had OSA.[20] This group had a higher apnea–hypopnea index and more of a tendency to be overweight or obese.

The potential for atherosclerosis is also greater among OSA patients.[21] Although these patients may be free of signs and symptoms of cardiovascular disease, atherosclerosis and coronary heart disease were found to be significantly higher as the degree of OSA worsened. The significance of this is critical if one considers that only 12.5% of a control group had signs of coronary heart disease while mild OSA patients demonstrated a 42% incidence and moderate to severe patients had an 80% incidence of disease in

**Table 5.1**  Risks for coronary heart disease relative to hours of sleep.

| Risk factor | Hours of sleep |
|---|---|
| 5 | 1.5–2 |
| 6 | 1–1.5 |
| 7–8 | 1 |
| 9+ | 1.5 or more |

*Source:* Adapted from Ayas NT. The adverse health effects of sleep restriction. Sleep Rev. 2003; (May/June):16.

multiple vessels.[22] Sleeping less than 7 hours a night or more than 8 hours may increase the risk for coronary heart disease (Table 5.1).

Endothelial dysfunction can also be associated with OSA. There can be subsequent relaxation in the vascular structures as well as atherosclerotic changes and cardiovascular disease, and the endothelial injury at a tissue level leads to atherogenesis.[23] The progression of atherosclerosis may be related to apnea events that alter inflammatory mediators and metabolic factors, which can result in hypertension.[24] These related events lead to atherosclerosis and cardiovascular disease.

A recent study has demonstrated that snoring alone may put patients at risk for atherosclerosis of the carotid artery.[25] The proposed mechanism involves vibrations in the pharyngeal airway that are in close proximity to the artery, and these vibrations may cause endothelial damage that results in inflammation and thereby promotes changes that may lead to atherosclerosis. The prevalence of the atherosclerosis worsened in direct proportion to the degree of snoring, and the prevalence ranged from 20% in mild snorers to 64% in heavy snorers.

### Congestive heart failure

The association of cardiovascular disease and sleep apnea is well known. CHF has been found to be prevalent in patients mainly with central sleep apnea (CSA).[26] The recurring respiratory events are associated with sleep disruption, arousals, hypoxia, and hypercapnia. It appears that a high percentage of patients with heart failure when screened for SRBD tested positive.[27] In addition, there is oftentimes a relation between Cheyne–Stokes respiration and CHF that is present in CSA patients.

Interestingly, the use of an oral appliance (OA) can beneficially impact CHF.[28,29] In these studies, the focus in determining the effect of OAs was based on the measurement of brain natriuretic peptide (BNP), which has been found to be elevated in OSA. This increase is linked to left ventricular pressure and volume levels. In patients with CHF, the BNP levels rise and are associated with sudden death, and it may predict morbidity and mortality.

### Cerebrovascular function and stroke

Stroke is the third leading cause of death and long-term disability.[30] The incidence of cerebrovascular disease and stroke is related to SRBD, and it is independent of other known risk factors for stroke.[31] The risk for stroke associated with OSA is also independent of hypertension, but the existence of hypertension, especially diurnal hypertension, further increases the risk. The mechanism is related to a decrease in cerebral perfusion and increased coagulation. There is an increased incidence of sudden death during sleep.[32] In addition, after a stroke, there is an increase in the prevalence of OSA, which affects the ability of the patient to rehabilitate and recover following the stroke.

### Triglycerides and cholesterol

HDL, or the good cholesterol, functions as both an antioxidant and antiatherogenic. HDL dysfunction has been found to be present in OSA patients.[33] This association is related to oxidative stress, which is present in patients with coronary heart disease. Lower levels of HDL have also been linked to issues with short-term memory deficits. Difficulty with memory has also been linked to OSA as one of the common symptoms.

## Diabetes type 2

2 diabetes is linked to SRBD such as snoring and OSA. In fact, snoring alone has been shown to be an independent risk factor for this type of diabetes.[34] The impact of snoring and OSA, by virtue of upper airway obstruction, may lead to oxygen desaturation that in turn may cause a rise in the level of cortisol and catecholamines. The outcome of this cascade may be an increase in insulin resistance, which is considered to be a precursor to diabetes. The Sleep Heart Health Study demonstrated that hypoxia during sleep resulted in glucose intolerance which was independent of age, sex, BMI, or the size of the waist.[1] Other studies have also shown that SRBD, irrespective of obesity, may serve as a contributing factor to diabetes through its association with glucose and insulin metabolism.[35–37]

Sleep disruption has also been shown to be common among those with type 2 diabetes.[38,39] Three main factors were found that are related to sleep disruption: obesity, pain, and an increase in the need to use the bathroom during the night. One-third of those who have type 2 diabetes experience sleep problems. In addition, the severity of the diabetes is directly related to the sleep disruption.

Sleep restrictions and excessive sleep are other issues that may impact the risk for diabetes (Table 5.2).[40] Getting between 7 and 8 hours of sleep a night is optimum. Less than 6–7 hours and over 8–9 hours may lead to an increased risk for diabetes.[1,41] After adjusting for BMI, where the tendency

**Table 5.2**  Risks for symptomatic diabetes relative to hours of sleep.

| Risk factor | Hours of sleep |
|---|---|
| 5 | 1.5–2 |
| 6 | 1–1.5 |
| 7–8 | 1 or < |
| 9+ | 1.5 or more |

*Source:* Adapted from Ayas NT. The adverse health effects of sleep restriction. Sleep Rev. 2003; (May/June):16.

for being overweight or obese was corrected, the increased risk for diabetes became modest (Table 5.2).

## Gastroesophageal reflux disease

Gastroesophageal reflux disease (GERD) (Table 5.3) is estimated in the United States to be experienced daily by 7% of the adult population and weekly by 70%.[42] Until more recently, though, there has been a slow acknowledgement of sleep-related GERD as well as its impact on daily function.[43]

Many people who have SRBD also may complain or may have been diagnosed with GERD.[44] The prevalence of GERD is much higher in patients with OSA as compared to the general population.[45] This is a condition that is associated with the relaxation of the phreno-esophageal sphincter where the esophagus enters the stomach, and it is oftentimes associated with obesity and diabetes.

GERD may be more prevalent in SRBD because of the following:

1.  Negative pressure in the airway is associated with narrowing of the airway during inspiration, which also impacts the esophagus. This negative inspiratory (intrathoracic) pressure generated during apnea is not selective to the airway, and thus the esophagus is also affected.[46]

**Table 5.3**  Common symptoms of gastroesophageal reflux disease.

| | |
|---|---|
| Nocturnal awakenings | Noncardiac chest pain |
| Laryngopharyngitis | Bronchial asthma |
| Chronic bronchitis | Pulmonary aspiration |
| Chronic cough | Acidic damage to teeth |

*Source:* Adapted from Demeter P and Pap A. The relationship between gastroesophageal reflux disease and obstructive sleep apnea. J Gastroenterol. 2004; 39(9):815–820.

During expiration, the negative pressure is released, and the potential for reflux to occur is greater.

2. Lying in the prone position where the effects of gravity are negated increases the risk for reflux. For this reason, many people with GERD sleep in an elevated position.

In like manner, GERD, particularly when present at night along with OSA, was found to be a cause of sleep disturbance.[47] The presence of GERD-type symptoms is also associated with awakenings from sleep. It has been estimated that the symptoms of GERD can cause awakenings in 58.6% of these patients.[48] Other symptoms associated with these awakenings are difficulty in initiating sleep and experiencing nightmares. It was also demonstrated that patients with GERD had more symptoms of excessive daytime sleepiness (EDS) as well.[49]

## Asthma

The presence of asthma, along with other respiratory conditions, may be associated with SRBD. In the general population, the prevalence of asthma is 5%. The coexistence of asthma and OSA is not well documented, although from a clinical perspective, many people who have SRBD also have asthma.

The one significant association that exists between asthma and SRBD is between asthma and GERD, the common denominator being the presence of inflammation. This same inflammatory condition has also been implicated in the progression of OSA. Nocturnal GERD associated with OSA can lead to the presentation of asthma.[50] The presence of airway obstruction and obesity are also common findings. The role of reflux in the precipitation of asthma has been linked to an elevation in BMI. As the BMI increases and obesity is more prevalent, the incidence of asthma also increases.

## Alzheimer's disease

The link between OSA and Alzheimer's disease is becoming more apparent. The common finding at this time is the presence of a genotypic marker known as apolipoprotein (APOE4), which is a risk factor for Alzheimer's and cardiovascular disease.[51] For those who carry this marker, there appears to be some complex interaction with brain pathology, cardiovascular disease, and OSA. One study demonstrated the relationship that exists between this genotype and OSA.[52]

OSA and the association of hypoxia in the elderly may be linked to mental deterioration that is associated with dementia.[53] In the future, more research will be needed to confirm this association, but the proper management of SRBD may be a significant factor. It is also plausible that the proper management of hypertension, elevated cholesterol, or diabetes, all three of which are three commonly occurring conditions in SRBD, can impact brain function.[54]

**Table 5.4** Oxidative stress: pathway to cardiovascular disease and atherosclerosis.

OSA—Episodic Hypoxia
Hypoxia/Reoxidation
⇓
ROS (Reactive Oxygen Species) – (increased)
⇓
Lymphocyte Activation
⇓
Adhesion Molecule Expression (increased)
⇓
Monocyte—Lymphocyte/Endothelial Adhesion (increased)
⇑ ⇓
⇓Nitric Oxide ⇐⇐Endothelial Dysfunction
⇓
Vascular Disease

*Source:* Adapted from Lavie L. Obstructive sleep apnoea syndrome—oxidative stress disorder. Sleep Med Rev. 2003; 7(1):35–51.

## Oxidative stress

Until the early part of the 2000s, the association of elevated blood pressure, cardiovascular disease, and other health issues as a consequence of SRBD, particularly snoring and OSA, were thought to be related to the presence of respiratory events during sleep. The significance of hypoxia associated with the drop in oxygen saturation was also a consideration as was the impact on the sympathetic nervous system.

The hypoxia that may occur during SRBD can lead to an increase in the prevalence of oxidative stress that in turn will lead to an increase in free radical production. This complicated group of events is directly linked to the presentation of cardiovascular disease, hypertension, and endothelial cell damage. There is an associated increase in what has been termed reactive oxygen species that is related to inflammation, erythropoietin (a protein that promotes red blood cell production), and adhesion molecules.[55] All these findings are associated with the presentation of the aforementioned cardiovascular consequences. In addition, there is a diminished level of nitric oxide, which is an agent that causes vascular relaxation or dilation and is itself a free radical. Levels of nitric oxide are impacted by hypoxia, particularly when the hypoxia is chronic.

A simplified flow diagram shows the impact of OSA and how hypoxia can lead to endothelial dysfunction and contribute to the presentation of cardiovascular disease. What can be seen is the presentation of inflammatory conditions that are implicated in both OSA and cardiovascular disease (Table 5.4).

In addition, the presentation of atherosclerosis may be an outcome of the modification of LDL (the bad cholesterol that contributes to the clogging of arteries) by oxidation that results in injury to endothelial cells as well as the underlying smooth muscle cells.

One animal study found that residual sleepiness, which may be an issue with some OSA patients despite adequate management of the apnea, may be related to long-term intermittent hypoxia associated with oxidative stress that results in neuronal injury of wake-promoting areas of the brain.[56] It is not clear as to what extent this gradual development may progress and to what degree the injury occurs. Additional study is needed to resolve this issue. However, the underlying thought may be that the sooner the SRBD is recognized and treated, the better off the outcome may be. To date, the treatment utilizes medication to manage the residual sleepiness.

# PAIN AND SLEEP

Pain and painful conditions can be worsened by the lack of sleep or by sleep disorders. In like manner, pain can lead to poor quality of sleep, a loss of sleep, and a reduction in an adequate number of hours of sleep that only continues to perpetuate the pain cycle. Thus, the improvement in sleep can in and of itself lead to pain reduction. This realization, despite the recognition of the relationship of these two conditions, has not had significant attention until recently.[57]

Studies have demonstrated that chronic pain can be present in 11–29% of the adult population,[58] and that 50–90% of these individuals can indicate that their sleep is adversely affected by their pain.[59–62]

There are a number of painful conditions that the dentist will encounter. As such, it is imperative that the loss or lack of sleep be considered in the overall management plan for the painful condition. In addition, it is essential that an understanding of the relationship between pain and its relationship to the sleep state be considered when planning for the management of each situation and condition.

# SLEEP BRUXISM

Many times the management of bruxism is predicated on tooth wear or co-existing conditions such as headache, myofascial pain (MFP), or temporomandibular disorders (TMD). It is important for the dentist to understand that bruxism is a sleep disorder as described in the *ICSD-2* classification of sleep disorders as well as in other resources.[63,64]

Sleep bruxism, also referred to as rhythmic masticatory muscle activity (RMMA), has been determined to be part of a sleep arousal response that is associated with the central nervous system and specifically the dopamine system.[65] Other factors have been considered such as psychological factors, stress, and personality traits, although they are now believed to play only a

**Table 5.5** Comparison of awake and sleep time bruxism.

| Awake time bruxers | Sleep time bruxers |
| --- | --- |
| Tooth clenching | Tooth grinding |
| Tooth tapping | Jaw muscle contractions |
| | Phasic (rhythmic) |
| Jaw bracing (no tooth contact) | Tonic (sustained) |

Source: Adapted from Roehrs JD. Sleep talking and noisy grinding. J Clin Sleep Med. 2006; 2(4):477–478.

minor role. In addition, other factors such as occlusion and other anatomic structures of the orofacial region that have in the past been considered to be factors in bruxism are now viewed as playing only a limited role.[66]

Sleep bruxism predominately occurs during nonrapid eye movement (NREM) stage 2 and rapid eye movement (REM) sleep.[67] There is also a relationship involving autonomic nervous system activity that precipitates tachycardia in association with the bruxing event. One study reported (1) that 4 seconds prior to the bruxing event, there was an increase in electroencephalographic (EEG) activity; (2) that one heartbeat prior to masticatory muscle depressor activity, there was a tachycardia; and (3) that within 800 milliseconds, there was masticatory muscle elevator activity.[68] All these reported events appear to be related to microarousals.

Another study demonstrated that with sleep bruxism, RMMA is present in about 60% of patients when asleep.[69] This is a slow movement of the orofacial structures that can become extreme in nature and lead to sleep bruxism. In addition, the resulting sleep bruxism may be more prevalent when the patient sleeps on their back.

Sleep bruxism was originally classified as a parafunctional activity that occurred during sleep. In the revised *ICSD-2*, sleep bruxism is viewed as a movement disorder and its classification is within the same category as restless legs syndrome (RLS) and periodic limb movement disorder (PLMD). Many times during a sleep study, the presence of RLS or PLMD activities is also found in sleep bruxers. Snoring and OSA have an increased risk in patients with sleep bruxism. It has been determined that the odds ratio for snoring, OSA, and EDS is 1.8, 1.4, and 1.3, respectively.[70]

Sleep bruxism may be classified as either a comparison of awake time versus sleep time or as primary versus secondary (Tables 5.5, 5.6, and 5.7).

# OROFACIAL PAIN

Of particular interest to the dentist are those patients that present with an orofacial pain condition. As with pain in general, these conditions are frequently associated with some type of sleep disruption. Similar to other

**Table 5.6**  Differentiation of primary and secondary bruxism.

| Primary (idiopathic) | Secondary (iatrogenic) |
| --- | --- |
| No known medical or dental causes | Associated with a medical or psychiatric condition |
| Exacerbated by psychosocial factors at times | Iatrogenic: following drug intake or withdrawal |

*Source:* Adapted from Kato T, Thie NMR, Montplaisir JY, et al. Bruxism and orofacial movements during sleep. In: Attanasio R and Bailey DR, eds. Sleep Disorders: Dentistry's Role. Dental Clinics of North America, 45. 2001; 657–684.

types of painful conditions, it may be difficult to determine which came first, the pain or the sleep problem.

Regardless of the type of orofacial pain complaint, addressing the sleep issues is most often helpful in managing the pain problem.

**Table 5.7**  Classification of secondary (iatrogenic) bruxism.

Movement disorders
  Oromandibular dyskinesia
  Oral tardive dyskinesia
  Huntington's disease
Neurologic or psychiatric disorders
  Dementia, depression, mental retardation
  Coma
  Cerebellar hemorrhage
Sleep-related disorders
  RLS and PLMD
  Apnea/snoring
  REM sleep behavior disorder
Chemical substances
  Alcohol
  Nicotine (smoking)
  Caffeine
  Cocaine
Medications
  Amphetamines
  Antipsychotic drugs
  Antidepressant drugs (especially selective serotonin reuptake inhibitors)
  Calcium blockers
  Antiarrhythmic drugs

*Source:* Adapted from Lavigne, GJ, Manzani C, and Kato T. Sleep bruxism. In: Kryger MH, Roth T, and Dement WC, eds. P and Practice of Sleep Medicine. 2005; 946–959.

## Myofascial pain

Muscle pain is a common finding among patients with poor sleep. However, not all patients with poor sleep will have muscle pain or muscle tenderness when palpated. Those with preexisting muscle pain are more likely to have insomnia as opposed to SRBD. Sleep disturbance is a common finding in MFP patients.[71] However, patients who snore or have OSA may also have muscular pain.

In some instances, muscle pain will not be restricted to just the orofacial structures, and it will encompass the entire body. These patients may be diagnosed with fibromyalgia (FM), a condition that is closely linked to sleep disruption as well as poor sleep quality and nonrestorative sleep.[72] One study demonstrated that greater than 50% of subjects diagnosed with FM also experienced chronic fatigue.[73] The FM patient will have the presence of multiple tender points that have been anatomically mapped, and the presence of these is a factor in determining the risk for this condition. MFP and FM are related, and their coexistence as well as the relationship to sleep disorders is important to recognize.

## Temporomandibular disorders

Many times the presence of TMD is associated with muscle pain and/or sleep bruxism. The occurrence of TMD in conjunction with poor sleep may be associated with MFP and/or bruxism that occurs during sleep and/or waking hours.

In 2001 a National Heart, Lung, and Blood Institute workshop reported that patients with TMD were also at risk for cardiovascular and sleep-related consequences.[74] The findings of this workshop concluded that patients with TMD were similarly at risk for and predisposed to cardiovascular disease, including related conditions such as hypertension, heart failure, and stroke. The study also concluded that additional research is needed to actually understand the relationship that appears to exist amongst these conditions. However, there is current evidence to suggest support of these findings. Of interest is the evidence that suggests this relationship may be related to interactions in the central nervous system. These interactions may impact the presentation of TMD as well as alterations in sleep architecture.

## Trigeminal neuralgia

This particular facial neuralgia is paroxysmal in nature and is precipitated by function or touch. The attacks are often unilateral, and they are described as sharp or electric-like and usually brief and unpredictable. The interesting fact related to this pain and sleep relationship is that the attacks do not occur during sleep.[75]

## Glossopharyngeal neuralgia

Glossopharyngeal neuraligia is similar to trigeminal neuralgia in that the attacks are paroxysmal, unilateral, and can be sharp to electric-like. They typically involve the ear, throat, tongue, or tonsillar area. Also the pain is oftentimes caused by function or touch. The difference from trigeminal neuralgia, though, is that the pain may awaken the patient from sleep.

## Temporal arteritis

Also known as giant cell arteritis, this is a pain that often feels like a headache with throbbing around the area of the temporal artery.[76] The patient may have pain in the masticatory muscles associated with chewing. The pain will frequently be worse at night and may be exaggerated by resting the head on a pillow.[77] Because of the serious nature of this type of pain, immediate attention to the treatment should be initiated once it is diagnosed.

## Atypical (idiopathic) toothache or atypical odontalgia

This type of orofacial pain is what appears to the patient as being an odontogenic pain, but it is without any distinct or obvious dental pathology. The pain is typically more prevalent in the maxillary posterior teeth, and it does not resolve with the use of local anesthesia. Because the pain is continuous and a cause is frequently elusive, the patient may become depressed or have increased stress, which in turn may lead to insomnia.

Relative to sleep, these patients will usually report that they will awaken with this pain, but they do not awaken because of the pain. The treatment of this condition is generally responsive to a low-dose regimen of tricyclic antidepressant medication.

# SLEEP LOSS AND PAIN

Of interest is the finding that sleep loss, specifically 4 hours and REM-type sleep, is associated with hyperalgesia the following day.[78] There is a bidirectional relationship between the loss of sleep and pain; that is, the loss of sleep impacts pain levels, and pain levels can reduce the amount of sleep.

One study demonstrated that sleep is analgesic in nature.[79] In patients with osteoarthritis, improvement of sleep latency and sleep efficiency was analgesic when compared to control subjects.

# HEADACHE DISORDERS

Headache and sleep disorders are the most prevalent conditions seen in clinical practice. As with other painful conditions, headaches can be related to sleep disturbances. Also similar to other pain, the headaches frequently will not resolve unless the sleep disorder is also addressed. As such, sleep may both provoke as well as relieve headaches.[80]

In particular, chronic daily and morning headaches are indicators of a probable sleep disorder. These encompass SRBD, insomnia, circadian rhythm disorders, and parasomnias. The most frequently reported headaches that are related to a sleep disorder are migraine, cluster, and muscle tension-type.

Headache seems to be more common in snorers as compared to nonsnorers. Habitual snoring is also more prevalent in chronic daily headache patients than in those with episodic headache. Insomnia can lead to headache, and the severity of headache is related directly to the degree of insomnia. Because insomnia is the most common sleep complaint relative to sleep disorders, it is found to occur in one-half to two-thirds of headache patients.[81]

In cluster headache, the presence of OSA is 8.4 times that of the normal population.[82] When the patient is over 40 years of age and has an increased BMI, the odds ratio increases. Accordingly, the risk decreases with a lower BMI and when the patient is less than 40 years old.

In the *ICSD-2*, the most common headaches that are sleep-related are the following: cluster, migraine, tension-type, and paroxsymal hemicrania (Table 5.8). Of the patients who had headache, 53% were diagnosed with OSA.

# CONCLUSION

Sleep disorders may contribute to the presence of a large number of chronic medical disorders.[83] The resolution and management of the medical condition, pain, headache complaint, and orofacial pain problems may best be achieved with the comanagement of a sleep disorder when it is present. Therefore, uncovering the presence of a sleep disorder or simply improving the patient's sleep may be significant in the resolution of the original concern.

Being an astute clinician now translates into looking for any contributing factors that may impact the situation as well as the resolution of that condition. All too often, the sleep issue is not addressed, and this makes it more difficult, more frustrating for the patient and clinician alike, and less cost effective when the ultimate goal is to efficiently and effectively manage the patient as a whole person.

Once a sleep disorder is uncovered, the next step is the appropriate treatment with the clinician who is most capable of managing the patient.

**Table 5.8**  Types of headaches—relationship to sleep.

| Type of headache | Relevant findings |
|---|---|
| Migraine headache | May occur at night with stages 3 and 4 NREM sleep |
| | Occurs in 54% of narcoleptics |
| | May be provoked by sleep |
| | Common to sleep for relief (related to serotonin) |
| | Responds best to proper sleep hygiene |
| Cluster headache | Occurs predominately at night between 9 and 10 p.m. |
| | Linked to REM sleep |
| | Linked to sleeping late |
| Chronic paroxysmal hemicrania (CPH) | May be greater at night |
| | May wake the patient |
| | Considered variant of cluster |
| | Linked to REM sleep |
| | Responds to indomethacin (indocin) |
| Tension-type headache (headaches on awakening) | Becomes less with increased activity—disappears when awake and active |
| | Successful treatment of sleep apnea decreases the headaches |
| | Occurs with increased bruxism, alcohol, sinus inflammation |
| Hypnic headache | Prevalent in older people |
| | REM sleep-related disorder |
| | Appears with dreams |
| | Diffuse location |
| | Duration of 1–2 hours |
| | No migraine symptoms |
| | Responds to aspirin |
| | Prophylactic therapy: lithium, caeffine, indocin |

*Source:* Adapted from Kryger MH, Roth T, and Dement WC, eds. Principles and Practice of Sleep Medicine. Philadelphia: Elsevier/Saunders. 2005; 879–881.

However, there are times when simply making the patient aware of the co-existence of a sleep problem lends a great deal to the patient's ability to self-manage their sleep and thus improve their quality of life.

In instances where the painful condition is associated with SRBD and OA therapy is determined to be a treatment option, the appropriate selection of an OA that will also address the airway may be the best choice.

The resolution of the sleep problem, particularly OSA, may have a major impact on the overall pain as well.

# REFERENCES

1. Quan SF, Howard BV, Iber C, et al. The Sleep Heart Health Study: design, rationale, and methods. Sleep. 1997; 20(12):1077–1085.
2. Coughlin SR, Mawdsley L, Mugarza J, et al. Obstructive sleep apnoea is independently associated with an increased prevalence of metabolic syndrome. Euro Heart J. 2004; 25(9):735–741.
3. Friedlander AH, Weinreb J, Friedlander I, et al. Metabolic syndrome: pathogenesis, medical care and dental implications. JADA. 2007; 138(2):179–187.
4. National Heart, Lung, and Blood Institute, National Institute of Health. What is Metabolic Syndrome? Available at http://www.nhlbi. nih.gov/health/dci/Diseases/ms/ms_whatis.html. Accessed 2009.
5. Grunstein R. Endocrine disorders. In: Kryger MH, Roth T, and Dement WC, eds. Principles and Practice of Sleep Medicine. 4th ed. Philadelphia: Elsevier/Saunders. 2005; 1237–1245.
6. Katz I, Stradling J, Slutsky AS, et al. Do patients with obstructive sleep apnea have thick neck? Am Rev Respir Dis. 1990; 141(5 Pt 1):1228–1231.
7. Guardiano S, Scott J, Catesby Ware J, et al. The long-term results of gastric bypass on idexes of sleep apnea. Chest. 2003; 124(4):1615–1619.
8. Hasler G, Buysse DJ, Klaghofer R, et al. The association between short sleep duration and obesity in young adults: a 13-year prospective study. Sleep. 2004; 27(4):661–666.
9. Taheri S, Lin L, Austin D, et al. Short sleep duration is associated with reduced leptin, elevated ghrelin, and increased body mass index. PLoS Med. 2004; 1(3):210–217.
10. Horne J. Short sleep is a questionable risk factor for obesity and related disorders: statistical versus clinical significance. Biol Psychol. 2008; 77(3):266–276.
11. Sekine M, Yamagami T, Handa K, et al. A dose-response relationship between short sleeping hours and childhood obesity: results of the Toyama birth control cohort study. Child Care Health Dev. 2002; 28(2):163–170.
12. Chami H and Gottlieb DJ. Sleep duration and cardiovascular health. Int J Sleep Wakefulness. 2008; 1(4):156–165.
13. Carlson JT, Hedner JA, Ejnell H, et al. High prevalence of hypertension in sleep apnea patients independent of obesity. Am J Respir Crit Care Med. 1994; 150: 72–77.
14. Morrell MJ, Finn L, Kim H, et al. Sleep fragmentation, awake blood pressure, and sleep-disordered breathing in a population-based study. Am J Respir Crit Care Med. 2000; 162: 2091–2096.
15. Loredo JS, Ziegler MG, Ancli-Israel S, et al. Relationship of arousals from sleep to sympathetic nervous system activity and BP in obstructive sleep apnea. Chest. 1999; 116(3):655–659.

16. Young T, Finn L, Hla JM, et al. Snoring as part of a dose-response relationship between sleep-disordered breathing and blood pressure. Sleep. 1996; 19(10):S202–S205.

17. Sjöström C, Lindberg E, Elmasry A, et al. Prevalence of sleep apnoea and snoring in hypertensive men: a population-based study. Thorax. 2002; 57: 602–607.

18. Kryger MH, Roth T, and Dement WC. Principles and Practice of Sleep Medicine. Elsevier/Saunders. 2005; 1171–1172.

19. Gami AS, Pressman G, Caples SM, et al. Association of atrial fibrillation and obstructive sleep apnea. Circulation. 2004; 110(4):364–367.

20. Schäfer H, Koehler U, Ewig S, et al. Obstructive sleep apnea as a risk marker in coronary artery disease. Cardiology. 1999; 92: 79–84.

21. Dragler LF, Bortolotto LA, Lorenzi MC, et al. Early signs of atherosclerosis in obstructive sleep apnea. Am J Respir Crit Care Med. 2005; 172: 613–618.

22. Lu G, ZW X, Liu JN, et al. A study on the association of obstructive sleep apnea hypopnea syndrome with coronary atherosclerosis and coronary heart disease. Zhonghua Jie HE He Hu Xi Za Zhi. 2007; 30(3):178–181.

23. Mary SM, Hung-Fat T, Lam B, et al. Endothelial function in obstructive sleep apnea and response to treatment. Am J Respir Crit Care Med. 2004; 169: 348–353.

24. Tsioufis C, Thomopoulos K, Dimitriadis K, et al. The incremental effect of obstructive sleep apnoea syndrome on arterial stiffness in newly diagnosed essential hypertension subjects. J Hypertens. 2007; 25(1):141–146.

25. Lee SA, Amis TC, Byth K, et al. Heavy snoring as a cause of carotid artery atherosclerosis. Sleep. 2008; 31(9):1207–1213.

26. Carmona-Bernal C, Quintana-Gallego E, Villa-Gil M, et al. Brain natriuretic peptide in patients with congestive heart failure and central sleep apnea. Chest. 2005; 127(5):1667–1673.

27. Trupp RJ, Hardesty P, Osborne J, et al. Prevalence of sleep disordered breathing in a heart failure program. Congest Heart Fail. 2004; 10(5):217–220.

28. Eskafi M. Sleep apnoea in patients with stable congestive heart failure—an intervention study with a mandibular advancement device. Swed Dent J Suppl. 2004; 168: 1–56.

29. Eskafi M, Cline C, Nilner M, et al. Treatment of sleep apnea in congestive heart failure with a dental device. Sleep Breath. 2006; 10: 90–97.

30. Mohsenin V. Is sleep apnea a risk factor for stroke? A critical analysis. Minerva Med. 2004; 95(4):291–305.

31. Mohsenin V. Sleep-disordered breathing: implications in cerebrovascular disease. Prev Cardiol. 2003; 6(3):149–154.

32. Culebras A. Cerebrovascular disease and the pathophysiology of obstructive sleep apnea. Curr Neurol Neurosci Rep. 2007; 7(2):173–179.

33. Tan KCB, Chow W, Lam JCM, et al. HDL dysfunction in obstructive sleep apnea. Atherosclerosis. 2005; 184(2):377–382.

34. Al-Delaimy WK, Manson JE, Willett WC, et al. Snoring as a risk factor for type II diabetes mellitus: a prospective study. Am J Epidemiol. 2002; 155(5):387–393.

35. Punjabi NM, Shahar E, Redline S, et al. Sleep-disordered breathing, glucose intolerance and insulin resistance—The Sleep Heart Health Study. Am J Epidemiol. 2004; 160:521–530.

36. Punjabi NM, Sorkin JD, Katzel LI, et al. Sleep-disordered breathing and insulin resistance in middle-aged and overweight men. Am J Respir Crit Care Med. 2002; 165:677–682.

37. Meslier N, Gagnadoux F, Giraud P, et al. Impaired glucose-insulin metabolism in males with obstructive sleep apnea syndrome. Europ Respir J. 2003; 22:156–160.

38. Lamond N, Tiggemann M, and Dawson D. Factors predicting sleep disruption in type II diabetes. Sleep. 2000; 23(3):1–2.

39. Resnick HE, Redline S, Shahar E, et al. Diabetes and sleep disturbances: findings from the Sleep Heart Health Study. Diabetes Care. 2003; 26(3):702–709.

40. Ayas NT. The adverse health effects of sleep restriction. Sleep Rev. 2003; (May/June):16–20.

41. Gottlieb DJ, Punjabi NM, Newman AB, et al. Association of sleep time with diabetes mellitus and impaired glucose tolerance. Arch Int Med. 2005; 165(8):863–867.

42. Locke GR, Talley NJ, Fett SL, et al. Prevalence and clinical spectrum of gastroesophageal reflux: a population-based study in Olmsted County, Minnesota. Gastroenterology. 1997; 112:1448–1456.

43. Shaker R, Castell DO, Schoenfeld PS, et al. Nighttime heartburn is an under-appreciated clinical problem that impacts sleep and daytime function: the results of a Gallup survey conducted on behalf of the American Gastroenterological Association. Am J Gastroenterol. 2003; 98:1487–1493.

44. Fass R, Quan SF, O'Connor GT, et al. Predictors of heartburn during sleep in a large prospective cohort study. Chest. 2005; 127:1658–1666.

45. Zanation AM and Senior BA. The relationship between extraesophageal reflux (EER) and obstructive sleep apnea (OSA). Sleep Med Rev. 2005; 9: 453–458.

46. Demeter P and Pap A. The relationship between gastroesophageal reflux disease and obstructive sleep apnea. J Gastroenterol. 2004; 39(9):815–820.

47. Suganuma N, Shigedo Y, Adachi H, et al. Association of gastroesophageal reflux with weight gain and apnea, and their disturbance on sleep. Psychiatry Clin Neurosci. 2001; 55(3):255–256.

48. Bruley des Varnes S, Errieau G, and Tessier C. Two thirds of patients with gastroesophageal reflux have nocturnal symptoms: survey by 562 general practitioners of 36663 patients. Presse Med. 2007; 36(4 Pt 1):591–597.

49. Guda N, Parington S, Shaw MJ, et al. Unrecognized GERD symptoms are associated with excessive daytime sleepiness in patients undergoing sleep studies. Dig Dis Sci. 2007; 52(10):2873–2876.

50. Orr WC. Gastrointestinal functioning during sleep: a new horizon in sleep medicine. Sleep Med Rev. 2001; 5(2):91–101.

51. Kadotani H, Kadotani T, Young T, et al. Association between apolipoprotein E4 and sleep-disordered breathing in adults. JAMA. 2001; 285(22):2888–2890.

52. Bliwise DL. Sleep apnea, APOE4 and Alzheimer's disease 20 years and counting? J Psychosom Res. 2002; 53(1):539–546.

53. Bliwise DL, Yesavage JA, Tinklenberg JR, et al. Sleep apnea in Alzheimer's disease. Neurobiol Aging. 1989; 10(4):343–346.

54. Macey PM, Henderson LA, Macey KE, et al. Brain morphology associated with obstructive sleep apnea. Am J Respir Crit Care Med. 2002; 166: 1382–1387.

55. Lavie L. Obstructive sleep apnoea syndrome—oxidative stress disorder. Sleep Med Rev. 2003; 7(1):35–51.

56. Morrell MJ. Residual sleepiness in patients with optimally treated sleep apnea: a case for hypoxia-induced oxidative brain injury. Sleep. 2004; 27(2):194–201.

57. Lavigne G, Sessle BJ, Choinière M, et al. Sleep and Pain. Seattle: IASP Press. 2007.

58. Harstall C and Ospina M. How prevalent is chronic pain? Pain Clin Updates. 2003; 11:1–4.

59. Morin CM, Gibson D, and Wade J. Self-reported sleep and mood disturbance in chronic pain patients. Clin J Pain. 1998; 14(4):311–314.

60. Smith MT, Perlis ML, Smith MS, et al. Sleep quality and presleep arousal in chronic pain. J Behav Med. 2000; 13:1–13.

61. McCracken LM and Iverson GL. Disrupted sleep patterns and daily functioning in patients with chronic pain. Pain Res Manag. 2002; 7:75–79.

62. Pilowsky I, Crettenden I, and Townley M. Sleep disturbance in pain clinic patients. Pain. 1985; 23:27–33.

63. American Academy of Sleep Medicine. The International Classification of Sleep Disorders, Second Edition. Westchester, IL: American Academy of Sleep Medicine. 2005; 189–191.

64. Lavigne GJ, Manzani C, and Kato T. Sleep bruxism. In: Kryger MH, Roth T, and Dement WC, eds. Principles and Practice of Sleep Medicine. Philadelphia: Elsevier/Saunders. 2005; 946–959.

65. Lobbezoo F and Naeije M. Bruxism is mainly regulated centrally, not peripherally. J Oral Rehab. 2001; 28:1085–1091.

66. Clark GT and Adler RC. A critical evaluation of occlusal therapy: occlusal adjustment procedures. JADA. 1985; 110:743–750.

67. Bader GG, Kasmpe T, Tagdae T, et al. Descriptive physiologic data on a sleep bruxism population. Sleep. 1997; 20(11):982–990.

68. Kato T, Rompre P, Montplaisir JY, et al. Sleep bruxism: an oromotor activity secondary to micro-arousal. J Dent Res. 2001; 80(10):1940–1944.

69. Kato T, Thie NMR, Montplaisir JY, et al. Bruxism and orofacial movements during sleep. In: Attanasio R and Bailey DR, eds. Sleep Disorders:

Dentistry's Role (Dental Clinics of North America, 45:4). Philadelphia: Elsevier/Saunders. 2001; 657–684.

70. Ohayin MM, Li KK, and Guilleminault C. Risk factors for sleep bruxism in the general population. Chest. 2001; 119:53–61.

71. Travel JG and Simons DG. Myofascial Pain and Dysfunction: The Trigger Point Manual. Baltimore: Williams & Wilkins. 1983; 91.

72. Moldofsky HK. Disordered sleep in fibromyalgia and related myofascial facial pain conditions. In: Attanasio R and Bailey DR, eds. Sleep Disorders: Dentistry's Role (Dental Clinics of North America, 45:4). Philadelphia: Elsevier/Saunders. 2001; 701–713.

73. White KP, Harth M, Speechley M, et al. A general population study of fibromyalgia tender points in noninstitutionalized adults with chronic widespread pain. J Rheumatol. 2000; 27(11):2677–2682.

74. NHLBI Workshop. Cardiovascular and sleep-related consequences of temporomandibular disorders. Final Report. 2001.

75. Turp JC and Gobetti JP. Trigeminal neuralgia verses atypical facial pain. Oral Surg Oral Med Oral Pathol. 1996; 81:424–432.

76. Austin D, O'Donnell F, and Attanasio R. Temporal arteritis mimics TMJ/myofascial pain syndrome. Ohio Dental J. 1992; 66(1):44–46.

77. Raskin NH. Giant cell arteritis. In: Raskin NH, ed. Headache. New York: Churchill Livingston. 1988; 320.

78. Roehrs T, Hyde M, Blaisdell B, et al. Sleep loss and REM sleep loss are hyperalgesic. Sleep. 2006; 29(2):145–151.

79. Vitiello M, Rybarczyk B, and Stephanski E. Sleep as analgesic: improving sleep and pain in older patients. Sleep. 2007; 30:A103.

80. Rains JC, Poceta JS, and Penzien DB. Sleep and headaches. Curr Neurol Neurosci Rep. 2008; 8(2):167–175.

81. Rains JC and Poceta JS. Headache and sleep disorders: review and clinical implications for headache management. Headache. 2006; 46:1344–1361.

82. Nobre M, Leal A, and Filho P. Investigation into sleep disturbance of patients suffering from cluster headache. Cephalgia. 2005; 25(7):488–492.

83. Collop N. The effect of obstructive sleep apnea on chronic medical disorders. Cleve Clin J Med. 2007; 74(1):72–78.

# Section 2

## Assessment of the Sleep-Related Breathing Disorder Patient

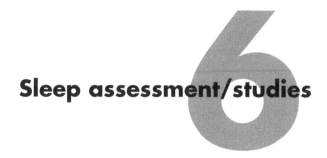

# Sleep assessment/studies

## CONCEPTUAL OVERVIEW

The *International Classification of Sleep Disorders, Second Edition (ICSD-2)* has classified 96 sleep disorders.[1] When a patient presents with chief concerns that are potentially related to sleep disorders, it may be necessary to augment the history-taking and clinical examination with subjective and/or objective measurement instruments in order to fully assess and diagnose the patient. These same measurement instruments have been beneficial when conducting research of sleep disorders.

Prior to when actual physiological information could be assessed via instrumentation, behavioral-based criteria were employed for descriptions of sleep.[2] The advent of laboratory-based polysomnographic studies allowed for the inclusion of measurable data regarding the physiological changes occurring during wake/sleep stages and disorders.[3]

The purpose of this chapter is to allow for the reader to understand the availability and application of different subjective-based self-assessment and objective-based assessments for sleep disorders.

## SUBJECTIVE SELF-ASSESSMENT

Relying on a patient to subjectively report his or her sleepiness without the use of a standardized set of questions is inconsistent and highly variable, especially with the significant potential to either underestimate or overestimate their sleepiness. At times it can be better to obtain a more consistent report from an individual who has the opportunity to observe that patient during sleep. However, this latter method is also flawed with its inherent inconsistencies since the patient's bed partner is generally not awake during the patient's entire sleep period to provide observable history that is consistent and accurate.

In an effort to quantify self-assessment of sleepiness, question-based instruments to subjectively estimate one's own sleepiness are composed of a standardized set of statements or questions. Although this type of self-assessment methodology does not provide objective physiologic data that measure wake/sleep periods of the patient, it does allow for a lower cost method to easily acquire at least some patient-based information that can be correlated with the patient's history and clinical examination.

## Epworth Sleepiness Scale

Of the available subjective-based self-assessments, the most frequently used instrument is the Epworth Sleepiness Scale (ESS), which was developed in 1991. The ESS has been demonstrated to identify degrees of sleepiness,[4] and the results are considered to be within acceptable limits for test–retest reliability.[5] The eight questions of the ESS query the individual about his or her subjective reporting of sleepiness relative to their expectation of dozing in eight different situations (Table 6.1).

In using a scale of 0–3, where 0 indicates no chance of dozing, 1 indicates a slight chance, 2 indicates a moderate chance, and 3 indicates a high chance, a total maximum score of 24 is possible. Investigations have shown that a score of 10 or 11 is considered to be the upper parameter for normal.[6,7] While higher scores correlate with sleep disorders, it has also been shown that scores also improve relative to the efficacy of management of sleep-related breathing disorders (SRBD).[8]

Although the ESS is attractive via its simplicity and ease of administration, the instrument does have its limitations, including not taking into account the individual's age, acuteness of sleep pathology, medical conditions, or use of pharmaceutics. Thus, the ESS is best when it is employed to be an adjunct to the patient history and clinical examination.

## Stanford Sleepiness Scale

Although not employed as commonly as the ESS, another self-assessment instrument is the Stanford Sleepiness Scale (SSS), which was developed in 1972.[9]

Through a questionnaire that utilizes a 7-point scale, the SSS provides a subjective measurement that relates to the individual's perception of sleepiness at a specific time (Table 6.2). It is regarded as a momentary evaluation and is therefore useful in assessing the degrees of perceived sleepiness throughout the period of a day. This ability to repeatedly be administered and reflect the current state of sleepiness is an advantage of the SSS over the ESS.

**Table 6.1**  Epworth Sleepiness Scale.

How likely are you to doze off or fall asleep in the
following situations, in contrast to just feeling tired?
This refers to your usual way of life in recent times. Even
if you have not done some of these things recently, try to
work out how they would have affected you. Use the following
scale to choose *the most appropriate number* for each
situation:

    0 = would never doze
    1 = slight chance of dozing
    2 = moderate chance of dozing
    3 = high chance of dozing

| Situation | Chance of dozing |
|---|---|
| Sitting and reading | ____ |
| Watching television | ____ |
| Sitting, inactive in a public place (e.g., theatre or meeting) | ____ |
| As a passenger in a car for an hour without a break | ____ |
| Lying down to rest in the afternoon when circumstances permit | ____ |
| Sitting and talking to someone | ____ |
| Sitting quietly after lunch without alcohol | ____ |
| In a car, while stopped for a few minutes in traffic | ____ |
| TOTAL | ____ |

*Source:* Adapted from Johns MW. A new method for measuring daytime sleepiness: the Epworth Sleepiness Scale. Sleep. 1991; 14:540–545.

As with the ESS, the inherent brevity of the SSS adds to the simplicity of administering it, although it is best when used to complement the patient history and clinical examination.

## OBJECTIVE-BASED ASSESSMENT

To definitively diagnose a sleep disorder, a complete collection of physiologic data from the wake/sleep stages needs to be obtained and interpreted. As defined by the American Academy of Sleep Medicine (AASM), there are four levels (I–IV) of sleep studies from which an objective-based assessment is made (Table 6.3).[10,11]. A level I study is regarded as the most accepted study for the assessment and treatment of obstructive sleep apnea (OSA). The four levels are differentiated per the number of simultaneously recorded physiological signals as well as whether or not the sleep study was attended by a sleep technologist.

**Table 6.2**    Stanford Sleepiness Scale.

Circle one number which best describes your level of
alertness or sleepiness right now.

| Scale | Characteristics |
|---|---|
| 1 | Feeling active and vital; wide awake |
| 2 | Functioning at a high level, but not at peak; able to concentrate |
| 3 | Relaxed; awake; not a full alertness; responsive |
| 4 | A little foggy, not at peak; let down |
| 5 | Fogginess; beginning to lose interest in remaining awake; slowed down |
| 6 | Sleepiness; prefer to be lying down; fighting sleep; woozy |
| 7 | Almost in reverie; sleep onset soon; lost struggle to remain awake |
| 8 | Asleep |

*Source:* Adapted from Hoddes E, Zarcone V, Smythe H, et al. Quantification of sleepiness: a new approach. Psychophysiology. 1973; 10:431–436.

## Polysomnography

A polysomnography (PSG) is an overnight sleep study attended by a sleep technologist during which at least seven different physiological signals are measured, and it is a level I study. The PSG is considered to be the "gold standard" in sleep medicine relative to objective-based sleep studies.[12] The

**Table 6.3**  Levels of sleep studies.

| | |
|---|---|
| Type I | A standard attended in-laboratory polysomnography (PSG) with a minimum of seven parameters measured (electroencephalogram—EEG; electrooculogram—EOG; chin electromyogram—EMG; electrocaradiogram—ECG; airflow; respiratory effort; oxygen saturation). |
| Type II | A comprehensive portable PSG that usually measures the same parameters as Type I, but it can be unattended. |
| Type III | Also referred to as a cardiorespiratory sleep study. A modified portable sleep apnea testing with a minimum of four parameters measured (heart rate or ECG, oxygen saturation, and at least two channels of respiratory movement or respiratory movement and airflow) and it is unattended. |
| Type IV | A continuous or dual bioparameter recording with a minimum of one parameter measured (oxygen saturation, flow, or chest movement) and it is unattended. |

*Source:* Adapted from Kushida CA, Littner MR, Morgenthaler TM, et al. Practice parameters for the indications for polysomnography and related procedures: an update for 2005. Sleep. 2005; 28(4):499–519.

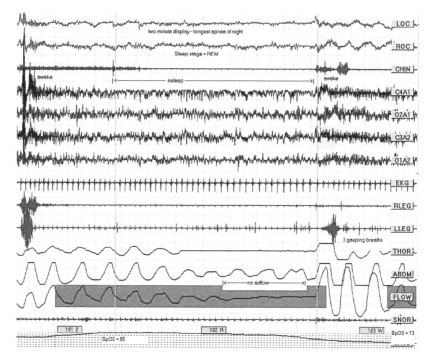

**Figure 6.1**    Attended polysomnograph demonstrating sleep apnea.

study is usually conducted in a sleep laboratory/center type of facility with trained staff to ensure proper placement of the necessary sensors as well as recognizing and addressing any displacement of sensors as needed during the study.[13]

The physiologic parameters measured during a PSG include simultaneous and continuous monitoring of at least brain wave activity, eye movements, muscle activity of the legs and mandible, body position, heart rate and rhythm, blood pressure, snoring, and respiratory activity that includes breathing patterns and oxygen saturation. Analysis of the data from these various measurements can reveal sleep disorder activities such as apneic events (Figure 6.1), hypopneic events (Figure 6.2), bruxism (Figure 6.3), snoring (Figure 6.4), and Cheyne–Stokes breathing (Figure 6.5).

A summary of the entire PSG data can be reflected in a graphic form called a hypnogram (Figure 6.6), which provides a comprehensive glimpse of sleep architecture relative to stages of sleep.

The raw data are scored into different sleep stages and physiologic activities in accordance with standardized criteria,[14] and a sleep physician interprets the study results, reviews the patient history and clinical examination data, and subsequently prepares a sleep study report of outcomes and recommendations. Most common sleep disorders can be assessed with a PSG,[15] including SRBD.[16] Effectiveness of treatment methods can also be achieved with a PSG.

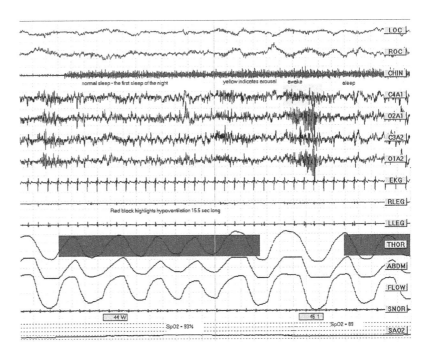

**Figure 6.2**   Attended polysomnograph demonstrating hypopnea.

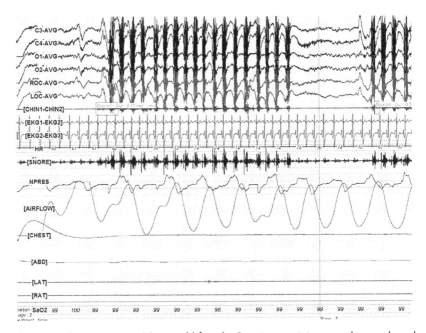

**Figure 6.3**   Bruxism in 29-year-old female. Prominent gritting sounds were heard on video replay. (Kakkar R and Hill G. Interpretation of the adult polysomnogram. Otolaryngol Clin North Am. 2007; 40(3):732. Reprinted with permission.)

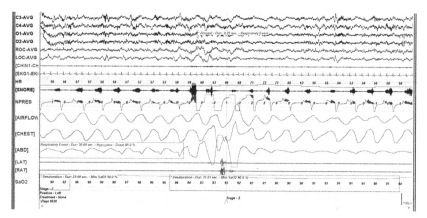

**Figure 6.4**   Snoring during a hypopnea. (Kakkar R and Hill G. Interpretation of the adult polysomnogram. Otolaryngol Clin North Am. 2007; 40(3):733. Reprinted with permission.)

Because the PSG is labor intensive and its complexity necessitates specialized facilities, equipment, and staff, most communities in the United States either do not have the availability to provide such testing or cannot meet the demand in a timely fashion.[17-20] This issue can be of particular concern since third-party payers require a PSG-based diagnosis for SRBD. For example, OSA on an annual basis necessitates a minimum of 2,310 PSG studies per 100,000 population to meet the current demand, yet

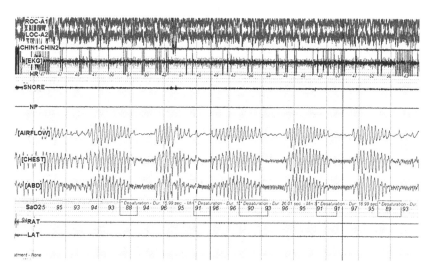

**Figure 6.5**   Cheyne–Stokes breathing. Note characteristic crescendo and decrescendo pattern in breathing effort, paralleling the airflow. (Kakkar R and Hill G. Interpretation of the adult polysomnogram. Otolaryngol Clin North Am. 2007; 40(3):736. Reprinted with permission.)

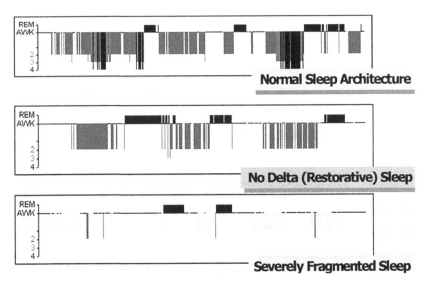

**Figure 6.6**    Hypnogram. (Kakkar R and Hill G. Interpretation of the adult polysomnogram. Otolaryngol Clin North Am. 2007; 40(3):727. Reprinted with permission.)

only 427 PSG studies per 100,000 population are conducted annually on the average.[21]

## Multiple Sleep Latency Test

A Multiple Sleep Latency Test (MSLT) is commonly used to measure daytime sleepiness.[8,22–24] The MSLT consists of a series of four to five 20-minutes daytime naps during 2-hour intervals at a sleep laboratory/center, and the test often lasts 7–8 hours. In addition, the test is to begin 1.5–3 hours after awakening from an overnight PSG. Similar to the PSG, sensors are placed by a trained sleep technologist in order to measure brain wave activity, eye movements, muscle activity of the mandible, and cardiac activity. There are standardized conditions under which the MSLT is performed,[25–27] including the instruction to the patient, "Please lie quietly, assume a comfortable position, keep your eyes closed, and try to fall asleep."

The physiological data outcomes demonstrate the amount of time it takes for the individual to initiate sleep (i.e., sleep latency) and to attain the different stages of sleep during each nap. The final scoring for the MSLT is the averaged times of sleep latency for the series of naps. An MSLT score of greater than 10 minutes is considered normal and less than 5 minutes is regarded as generally indicating the presence of a sleep disorder. Individuals who demonstrate a quick onset of rapid eye movement sleep are also more likely to have a sleep disorder.

**Table 6.4**  Indications for the use of the Multiple Sleep Latency Test (MSLT).

| | |
|---|---|
| 1 | The MSLT is indicated as part of the clinical evaluation for patients with suspected narcolepsy to confirm the diagnosis. |
| 2 | The MSLT may be indicated as part of the evaluation of patients with suspected idiopathic hypersomnia to help differentiate hypersomnia from narcolepsy. |
| 3 | The MSLT is not routinely indicated in the initial evaluation and diagnosis of obstructive sleep apnea syndrome or in assessment of change following treatment with nasal continuous positive airway pressure (CPAP). |
| 4 | The MSLT is not routinely indicated evaluation of sleepiness in medical and neurological disorders (other than narcolepsy), insomnia, or circadian rhythm disorders. |
| 5 | Repeat MSLT testing may be indicated in the following situations: (1) when the initial test is affected by extraneous circumstances or when appropriate study conditions were not present during initial testing, (2) when ambiguous or uninterpreted findings are present, and (3) when the patient is suspected to have narcolepsy but earlier MSLT evaluation(s) did not provide polygraphic confirmation. |

*Source:* Adapted from Standards of Practice Committee of the American Academy of Sleep Medicine. Practice parameters for clinical use of the multiple sleep latency test and the maintenance of wakefulness test. Sleep. 2005; 28(1):113–121.

Often the MSLT is the instrument of choice to definitively diagnose narcolepsy or idiopathic hypersomnia. The MSLT can also be used to document outcomes of treatment.[28–30] Residual sleepiness can also be demonstrated for those individuals who do not report sleepiness after undergoing treatment.[31]

In and of itself, the MSLT is not regarded as an accurate means to differentiate pathologic sleep disorders. Practice parameters for the clinical application of the MSLT have been published by the AASM.[27,32] Table 6.4 identifies specific indications for the use of the MSLT from the AASM report.

## Maintenance of Wakefulness Test

A Maintenance of Wakefulness Test (MWT) is commonly used to measure the alertness of an individual during the waking hours.[33] The MWT can also be employed to assess a sleep disorder patient's response to treatment. Whereas the MSLT determines whether or not an individual can initiate sleep sooner than what is regarded as a normal amount of time, the MWT determines whether or not an individual can stay awake for what is regarded as a normal amount of time.

Similar to the MSLT, sensors are placed by a trained sleep technologist in order to measure brain wave activity, eye movements, muscle activity of the mandible, and cardiac activity, and subsequently there is a series

**Table 6.5**  Indications for the use of the Maintenance of Wakefulness Test (MWT).

| | |
|---|---|
| 1 | The MWT 40-minute protocol may be used to assess an individual's ability to remain awake when his or her inability to remain awake constitutes a public or personal safety issue. |
| 2 | The MWT may be indicated in patients with excessive sleepiness to assess response to treatment. |

*Source:* Adapted from Portable Monitoring Task Force of the American Academy of Sleep Medicine. Clinical guidelines for the use of unattended portable monitors in the diagnosis of obstructive sleep apnea in adult patients. J Clin Sleep Med. 2007; 3(7):737–747.

of four to five 20-minute daytime naps during 2-hour intervals at a sleep laboratory/center.[33] Although there are also similar standardized conditions under which the MWT is performed,[25–27] the significant procedural difference of the MWT from the MSLT is with the instruction to the patient, "Please sit still and remain awake for as long as possible. Look directly ahead of you, and do not look directly at the light."[27,34]

The physiological data outcomes demonstrate the ability of an individual to stay awake. The final scoring for the MWT is the averaged times of wakefulness for the series. An MWT score of 8 minutes or more is considered normal, whereas abnormal would be an average of initiating sleep in less than 8 minutes. If the individual does not fall asleep in 40 minutes, then the test is terminated.

Practice parameters for the clinical application of the MSLT have been published by the AASM.[27,32] Table 6.5 identifies specific indications for the use of the MWT from the AASM report.

With a heightened awareness in sleep disorders relative to public safety, the MWT is acknowledged by the Federal Aviation Administration as a method of assessing effectiveness of treatment for excessive daytime sleepiness and thereby affording the ability to the Aviation Medical Examiners to reissue an airman medical certificate for commercial airline pilots.[35]

As with the other assessment instruments, test outcomes must be viewed in light of the patient history and clinical examination. Also, it has been shown that there is poor correlation between the ESS, MSLT, and MWT.[36–38]

# PORTABLE MONITORING DEVICES

The in-laboratory PSG is regarded as the current "gold standard" procedure for the evaluation of sleep and the diagnosis of SRBD, including but not limited to OSA, central sleep apnea, and Cheyne–Stokes breathing.[12] However, because of the associated high costs and issues of availability and accessibility of the PSG, there has been an increased interest in the use of portable monitoring (PM) devices as an alternative for the objective

**Table 6.6** Indications for portable monitoring (PM).

| | |
|---|---|
| 1 | PM for the diagnosis of obstructive sleep apnea (OSA) should be performed only in conjunction with a comprehensive sleep evaluation. Clinical sleep evaluations using PM must be supervised by a practitioner with board certification in sleep medicine or an individual who fulfills the eligibility criteria for the sleep medicine certification examination. In the absence of a comprehensive sleep evaluation, there is no indication for the use of PM. |
| 2 | Provided that the recommendations of #1 have been satisfied, PM may be used as an alternative to polysomnography (PSG) for the diagnosis of OSA in patients with a high pretest probability of moderate to severe OSA. PM should not be used in the patient groups with comorbid medical conditions (e.g., severe pulmonary disease, neuromuscular disease, or congestive heart failure), other sleep disorders (e.g., central sleep apnea, periodic limb movement disorder, insomnia, parasomnias, circadian rhythm disorders, or narcolepsy), or for general screening of asymptomatic patients. |
| 3 | PM may be indicated for the diagnosis of OSA in patients for whom in-laboratory PSG is not possible by virtue of immobility, safety, or critical illness. |
| 4 | PM may be indicated to monitor the response to non-CPAP treatments for OSA, including oral appliances, upper airway surgery, and weight loss. |

*Source:* Adapted from Portable Monitoring Task Force of the American Academy of Sleep Medicine. Clinical guidelines for the use of unattended portable monitors in the diagnosis of obstructive sleep apnea in adult patients. J Clin Sleep Med. 2007; 3(7):737–747.

assessment of sleep as well as for measuring effectiveness of treatment for SRBD. Some studies state that PM devices can collect the same data as in-laboratory PSG.[39,40]

In 1994, the AASM published its first practice parameters for the use of PM in assessing OSA.[41] A review of the literature and evidence regarding ambulatory testing with PM devices was performed by the AASM,[42] and a subsequent practice parameters report regarding the use of PM devices relative to OSA was published in 2003.[43] The most recent AASM guidelines for the clinical use of PM devices in assessing individuals suspected of having OSA were published in 2007.[12] Table 6.6 identifies specific indications for the use of PM devices from the 2007 AASM report. Specific indication #4 will be of interest to the dentist treating OSA patients with oral appliance (OA) therapy since PM devices may provide valuable follow-up objective documentation to supplement the patient's subjective documentation relative to the effectiveness of OA therapy:

This recommendation is based on Task Force consensus. PM may be used to monitor the efficacy of therapies other than CPAP when the diagnosis of OSA has already been made, either through PM or in-laboratory PSG.[12]

Up to this point, unless an OSA patient has undergone an in-laboratory PSG subsequent to the use of an OA, the only acceptable documentation for therapeutic effectiveness has been the subjective responses of the patient and/or the patient's bed partner.

## CONCLUSION

Because of the multitude of categories of sleep disorders and the serious and life-threatening conditions of some of these disorders, it is typical for the evaluation process to include subjective and/or objective measurement instruments in order to obtain a complete assessment of the patient. There are various diagnostic modalities and instruments available. A subjective-based questionnaire-type of instrument may be useful for the practitioner to make appropriate clinical predictions. There are also in-laboratory sleep studies that may provide more comprehensive physiological assessments to assist in determining the diagnosis and appropriate management plan.

The dentist has an opportunity to be an integral component in the screening and management process for SRBD. In order to do so, it is prudent for the dentist to be familiar with the various diagnostic instruments and modalities available for sleep assessment.

## REFERENCES

1. Hauri PJ, Task Force Chair. International Classification of Sleep Disorders, Second Edition. Westminster, IL: American Academy of Sleep Medicine. 2005.
2. Tobler I. Is sleep fundamentally different between mammalian species? Behav Brain Res. 1995; 69:35.
3. Zee PC and Turek FW. Introduction to sleep and circadian rhythms. In: Turek FW and Zee PC, eds. Regulation of Sleep and Circadian Rhythms. New York: Marcel Dekker Inc. 1999; 1–17.
4. Johns MW. A new method for measuring daytime sleepiness: the Epworth Sleepiness Scale. Sleep. 1991; 14:540–545.
5. Johns MW. Sleepiness in different situations measured by the Epworth Sleepiness Scale. Sleep. 1994; 17:703–710.
6. Johns MW and Hocking B. Daytime sleepiness and sleep habits of Australian workers. Sleep. 1997; 20:844–849.
7. Parkes JD, Chen SY, Clift SJ, et al. The clinical diagnosis of the narcoleptic syndrome. J Sleep Res. 1998; 7:41–52.
8. Redline S, Adams N, Strauss ME, et al. Improvement of mild sleep-disordered breathing with CPAP compared with conservative therapy. Am J Respir Crit Care Med. 1998; 157:858–865.
9. Hoddes E, Zarcone V, Smythe H, et al. Quantification of sleepiness: a new approach. Psychophysiology. 1973; 10:431–436.

10. Kushida CA, Littner MR, Morgenthaler TM, et al. Practice parameters for the indications for polysomnography and related procedures: an update for 2005. Sleep. 2005; 28(4):499–519.

11. Ferber R, Millan R, Coppoloy M, et al. American Sleep Disorders Association: portable recording in assessment of obstructive sleep apnea. Sleep. 1994; 17:378–392.

12. Portable Monitoring Task Force of the American Academy of Sleep Medicine. Clinical guidelines for the use of unattended portable monitors in the diagnosis of obstructive sleep apnea in adult patients. J Clin Sleep Med. 2007; 3(7):737–747.

13. American Sleep Disorders Association. Role and Qualifications of Technologists Performing Polysomnography: Position Paper. Adopted by the Executive Committee of the American Sleep Disorders Association. April 1, 1998.

14. Rechtschaffen A and Kales A. A Manual of Standardized Terminology, Techniques, and Scoring Systems for Sleep Stages of Human Subjects. Bethesda: National Institute of Neurological Disease and Blindness. 1968.

15. Ross SD, Sheinhait IA, Harrison KJ, et al. Systematic review and meta-analysis of the literature regarding the diagnosis of sleep apnea. Sleep. 2000; 23:519–532.

16. American Thoracic Society, Medical Section of the American Lung Association. Indications and standards for cardiopulmonary sleep studies. Am Rev Respir Dis. 1989; 139:559–568.

17. Banno K and Kryger MH. Factors limiting access to services for sleep apnea patients. Sleep Med Rev. 2004; 8(4):253–255.

18. Tachibana N, Ayas A, and White DP. A quantitative assessment of sleep laboratory activity in the United States. J Clin Sleep Med. 2005; 1(1): 23–26.

19. Rodsutti J, Hensley M, Thakkinstian A, et al. A clinical decision rule to prioritize polysomnography in patients with suspected sleep apnea. Sleep. 2004; 27(4):694–699.

20. Sharafkhaneh A, Richardson P, and Hirshkowitz M. Sleep apnea in a high risk population: a study of veterans health administration beneficiaries. Sleep Medicine. 2004; 5(4):345–350.

21. Flemons WW, Douglas NJ, Kuna ST, et al. Access to diagnosis and treatment of patients with suspected sleep apnea. Am J Resp Crit Care Med. 2004; 169(6):668–672.

22. Carskadon MA and Dement WC. Sleep tendency: an objective measure of sleep loss. Sleep Res. 1977; 6:200.

23. Richardson GS, Carskadon MA, Flagg W, et al. Excessive daytime sleepiness in man: multiple sleep latency measurement in narcoleptic and control subjects. Electroencephalogr Clin Neurophsysiol. 1978; 45:621–627.

24. Carskadon MA and Rechtschaffen AT. Monitoring and staging human sleep. In: Kryger M, Roth T, and Dement WC, eds. Principles and Practice of Sleep Medicine. 3rd ed. Philadelphia: WB Saunders. 2000; 1203–1206.

25. Carskadon MA, Dement WC, Mitler MM, et al. Guidelines for the multiple sleep latency test (MSLT): a standard measure of sleepiness. Sleep. 1986; 9:519–524.

26. Roehrs TA and Carskadon MA. Standardization of method: essential to sleep science. Sleep. 1998; 21:445.

27. Standards of Practice Committee of the American Academy of Sleep Medicine. Practice parameters for clinical use of the multiple sleep latency test and the maintenance of wakefulness test. Sleep. 2005; 28(1):113–121.

28. Dement WC, Carskadon MA, and Richardson GS. Excessive daytime sleepiness in the sleep apnea syndrome. In: Guilleminault C and Dement WC, eds. Sleep Apnea Syndromes. Menlo Park, CA: Alan R. Liss. 1978; 23–46.

29. Lamphere J, Roehrs T, Wittig R, et al. Recovery of alertness after CPAP in apnea. Chest. 1989; 96:1364–1367.

30. U.S. Modafinil in Narcolepsy Study Group (USMNSG). Randomized trial of modafinil for the treatment of pathological somnolence in narcolepsy. Ann Neurol. 1998; 43:88–97.

31. Zorick F, Roehrs T, Conway W, et al. Effects of unulopalatopharyngoplasty on the daytime sleepiness associated with sleep apnea syndrome. Bull Eur Physiopathol Respir. 1983; 19:600–603.

32. Littner MR, Kushida C, Wise M, et al. A review by the MSLT and MWT Task Force of the Standards of Practice Committee of the American Academy of Sleep Medicine: the clinical use of the MSLT and MWT. Sleep. 2005; 28:123–144.

33. Mitler MM, Gujavarty KS, and Browman CP. Maintenance of wakefulness test: a polysomnographic technique for evaluation of treatment efficacy in patients with excessive somnolence. Electroencephalogr Clin Neurophysiol. 1982; 53:658–661.

34. Doghramjii K, Mitler M, Sangal R, et al. A normative study of the maintenance of wakefulness test (MWT). Electroencephaloogr Clin Neurophysiol. 1997; 103:554–562.

35. Federal Aviation Administration (FAA). Guide for Aviation Medical Examiners Special Issuances. Available at www.faa.gov. Accessed January 9, 2008.

36. Johns MW. Sensitivity and specificity of the multiple sleep latency test (MSLT), the maintenance of wakefulness test, and the Epworth Sleepiness Scale: failure of the MSLT as a gold standard. J Sleep Res. 2000; 9:5–11.

37. Sangal RB, Mitler MM, and Sangal JM. Subjective sleepiness ratings (Epworth Sleepiness Scale) do not reflect the same parameter of sleepiness as objective sleepiness (maintenance of wakefulness test) in patients with narcolepsy. Clin Neurophysiol. 1999; 110:2131–2135.

38. Weaver TE. Outcome measurements in sleep medicine practice and research. Part I: assessment of symptoms, subjective and objective daytime sleepiness, health-related quality of life and functional status. Sleep Med Rev. 2001; 5:103–128.

39. Iber C, Redline S, Kaplan Gilpin AM, et al. Polysomnography performed in the unattended home versus the attended laboratory setting—Sleep Heart Health Study methodology. Sleep. 2004; 27(3):536–540.

40. Goodwin JL, Kaemingk KL, Fregosi RF, et al. Clinical outcomes associated with sleep-disordered breathing in Caucasian and Hispanic children—the Tucson Children's Assessment of Sleep Apnea Study (TuCASA). Sleep. 2003; 26(5):587–591.

41. Standards of Practice Committee of the American Academy of Sleep Medicine. Practice parameters for the use of portable recording in the assessment of obstructive sleep apnea. Sleep. 1994; 17:372–377.

42. Flemons WW, Littner MR, Rowley JA, et al. Home diagnosis of sleep apnea: a systematic review of the literature. An evidence review cosponsored by the American Academy of Sleep Medicine, the American College of Chest Physicians, and the American Thoracic Society. Chest. 2003; 124(4):1543–1579.

43. Chesson AL Jr, Berry RB, and Pack A. Practice parameters for the use of portable monitoring devices in the investigation of suspected obstructive sleep apnea in adults. Sleep. 2003; 26:907–913.

# Evaluation by the dentist

7

## CONCEPTUAL OVERVIEW

The dentist is called on today, more than ever, to be cognizant of related health care issues of their patients and not just of their dental and oral health status. This understanding and subsequent formal training in dental education began several decades ago with the recognition of hypertension when the blood pressure was taken at an initial visit or at a periodic visit for reevaluation, such as a dental hygiene visit. When the blood pressure was elevated, the patient was advised to contact their physician and have this evaluated more thoroughly. This heightened awareness led to the recognition of many people who were at risk for hypertension and who otherwise would have been undetected.

More recently, the association between periodontal disease and cardiovascular disease has been identified, and more aggressive steps are being taken clinically to resolve the periodontal condition in order to reduce the risk for cardiovascular disease. More than any other health care provider, oral cancer screening is another action that the dentist implements during the initial and follow-up care visits. Other examples are related to the recognition of oral conditions associated with systemic illnesses such as diabetes, leukemia, and many of the autoimmune diseases (e.g., Sjogren's syndrome).

Sleep disorders, and particularly obstructive sleep apnea (OSA), are no exception. Not only are sleep disorders prevalent in the general population, but they also have a potential for significant impact on an individual's health as well as on society. Sleep disorders may impair one's quality of life and daily performance relative to schooling, driving or operating any other machinery, the workplace, and relationships.

The role of the dentist in the recognition of patients at risk for OSA and other sleep-related breathing disorders (SRBD), such as snoring, is now well established. The dentist is just as likely to identify a patient who is at risk for OSA as is the physician.[1] However, a study found that dentists had a general deficiency in their ability to recognize a patient at risk for OSA, and they also knew very little about the use of oral appliance (OA) therapy for the management of SRBD.[2] Also, only an estimated 16% of the dentists were taught anything about SRBD in dental school, and about 40% knew very little about OA therapy for the management of OSA. The study demonstrated the need for more education related to OSA and the use of an OA as an option for the management of the patient diagnosed with OSA.

# WHAT THE DENTIST SEES THAT INDICATES THE RISK FOR SRBD

The dentist as well as the dental hygienist sees patients regularly who have signs of SRBD. However, unless the practitioner is knowledgeable of and recognizes the potential for these findings to suggest that there is a risk for SRBD, the sleep disorder may go undetected. Many of the conditions that may be identified by both the dentist and the dental hygienist that may indicate a risk for SRBD and health-related issues are commonly observed findings. Unfortunately, these findings often may be evaluated on their own merit as being stand-alone, and thus they may not be considered as potentially being related to some other health issue.

Once any of these conditions are recognized, then it becomes imperative to do the following: (1) determine if the risk for snoring or OSA is present, (2) inform the patient of the findings, and (3) consult with them regarding the appropriate measures needed for a complete diagnosis and management plan.

Many intra- and extraoral conditions have an association with risk for SRBD that warrant in-depth consideration (Table 7.1).

# ASKING THE PROPER QUESTIONS

The addition of a few questions to the existing health history questionnaire is an important element of the data collection phase. These questions may not only uncover an individual who is at risk for snoring or having OSA, but they may also assist in the identification of someone who has been previously diagnosed with SRBD.

**Table 7.1**  Conditions that indicate the risk for a sleep-related breathing disorder: sleep apnea and snoring.

| Observed condition | What this may indicate |
| --- | --- |
| Wear on the teeth | Indicative of sleep bruxism |
| Scalloped borders (crenations) of the tongue | Found to correlate with an increased risk for sleep apnea[12] |
| Enlarged tongue | Increased potential for upper airway obstruction |
| Coated tongue | Possible gastroesophageal reflux disease |
| Enlarged, swollen, or elongated uvula | Increased potential for snoring or sleep apnea |
| Large tonsils | Higher incidence of airway obstruction |
| Narrow airway | Greater risk for snoring or sleep apnea |
| Gingival recession and/or abfraction | Greater potential for sleep bruxism (grinding or clenching) |
| Tongue obstructs view of airway (Mallampati score) | The greater the obstruction, the higher the potential for snoring and sleep apnea |
| Chronic mouth breather (poor lip seal) | Blocked nasal airway; more likely to snore |

The basic questions that the dentist might include in the initial patient history form are the following:

- Do you or have you been told you snore when sleeping?
- Are you tired upon awakening from sleep or during the day?
- Do you fall asleep or are you drowsy in inappropriate situations such as in meetings, at movies, at church, or in social situations?
- Are you drowsy when driving?
- Do you have headaches in the morning?

If the response to any of these questions is positive, then additional questioning for a more comprehensive understanding of any potential sleep disorders may be necessary.

To further recognize a patient who may be at risk for OSA, the use of a common questionnaire known as the Epworth Sleepiness Scale (ESS) is utilized. The ESS identifies patients who are experiencing symptoms related to daytime sleepiness, which suggests the risk for OSA (Figure 7.1).[3] This eight-item survey can be easily completed by the patient, and the scored results assist the practitioner in considering the appropriate course of action that may be advisable, which, most often, is a referral for a sleep study (polysomnogram) or to the patient's physician for further evaluation.

Epworth Sleepiness Scale

| Situation | Chance of Dozing (0–3) | | | |
|---|---|---|---|---|
| Sitting and reading | 0 | 1 | 2 | 3 |
| Watching television | 0 | 1 | 2 | 3 |
| Sitting inactive (meeting, movie, church) | 0 | 1 | 2 | 3 |
| As a passenger in a car – for an hour – no break | 0 | 1 | 2 | 3 |
| Lying down to rest in the afternoon | 0 | 1 | 2 | 3 |
| Sitting and talking to someone | 0 | 1 | 2 | 3 |
| Sitting quietly after lunch (had no alcohol) | 0 | 1 | 2 | 3 |
| Stopped at a light or in traffic | 0 | 1 | 2 | 3 |
| | | | Total Score | |

0 = would never doze        2 = moderate chance of dozing
1 = slight chance ofdozing    3 = high chance ofdozing

**Figure 7.1** Epworth Sleepiness Scale—modified and adapted from original version. (Johns MW. A new method for measuring daytime sleepiness: the Epworth Sleepiness Scale. Sleep 1991; 14:540–545.)

Interpretation of the ESS score is a common means of communication within the sleep medicine field regarding the risk for OSA. As the total score approaches 9, the risk for OSA increases.[4] As the total score becomes greater than 9, then the risk factors are considered to be even more significant. An elevated score, though, is not always definitive for OSA and is also not indicative of its severity. The results from the ESS also need to be considered in light of other clinical and patient history findings.

The second portion of the ESS evaluates the patient's behavior during sleep and more specifically some of the well-recognized characteristics associated with OSA. Snoring and its severity are assessed along with conditions associated with snoring that may suggest an increased risk for OSA such as waking up gasping for air or experiencing a choking sensation during sleep. If snoring is the only recognized condition along with the ESS total score being less than 9, then the risk for OSA may be less, but this is not always the case.

# CLINICAL SCREENING FOR SRBD

Once it has been determined that a patient is at risk for SRBD, it may be advisable to perform a sleep disorder screening examination. In most instances, a significant amount of clinical information regarding the patient's dental and medical status and history has already been collected. The screening evaluation will supplement the existing record with documentation that is designed to identify relevant conditions that support the possible risk for SRBD, in particular for OSA.

Table 7.2 reflects the progression of steps that might be considered to assess the patient who is at risk for SRBD.

**Table 7.2**  Steps for assessment of the patient at risk for a sleep-related breathing disorder and sleep apnea.

| | |
|---|---|
| Step 1: | Recognition of existing risk factors (Table 7.1) |
| Step 2: | Positive response(s) to the health history questions |
| Step 3: | Completion of the Epworth Sleepiness Scale |
| Step 4: | Discussion with the patient regarding the positive responses from above |
| Step 5: | Reappointment for clinical screening evaluation |
| | Consultation to discuss findings |
| | Make recommendations for management plan |
| | Management options |
| | • Refer to patient's physician for further evaluation |
| | • Refer for a sleep study |

*Source:* Treatment Sequencing. Handout for the UCLA School of Dentistry Dental Sleep Medicine Mini-Residency; 2009.

There are a number of components that should make up an SRBD screening evaluation, including SRBD history, review of medical history, review of current medications, temporomandibular disorders (TMD) assessment, oral airway evaluation, nasal airway evaluation, and subjective airway testing.

## SRBD history

The SRBD history is designed to obtain patient's history-related findings that are specific to SRBD, such as the following patient symptoms or previously diagnosed conditions:

- Snoring
- Sleep apnea
- Low energy
- Daytime sleepiness/tired
- Difficult to concentrate
- Previous or current use of positive airway pressure therapy
- Previous surgery for SRBD
- Mood swings/irritable
- Feel depressed
- Headaches
- Bruxism (grinding and/or clenching)

## Review of medical history

The patient's medical history may be indicative of an underlying sleep issue. A number of preexisting medical conditions may suggest an increased risk for SRBD, particularly OSA, such as the following:

- Hypertension
- Cardiovascular disease

- Headaches
- Respiratory conditions (especially asthma)
- Diabetes
- Gastroesophagal acid reflux disease
- Hypothyroidism
- Allergy

## Review of current medications

The patient's current medications need to be reviewed. There may be prescription medicines that are being used for the management of a medical condition, yet the condition may be related to a sleep disorder. In addition, many medications may have an impact on the patient's sleep.

### Medications and sleep

Almost all medications that are taken can impact sleep in some manner. Table 7.3 outlines some of the more common medications that are frequently encountered in a dental practice and which may impact sleep.

Not all patients have similar responses to medications, and they may not experience an adverse effect on their sleep. Also, patients may be taking medications for a particular health issue, and this may also be an indicator that a sleep disorder is present but may have been overlooked or not considered. In addition, there are many medications that are used to promote and improve sleep.

**Medications by class associated with sleepiness**
*As reported in clinical trials and case reports*
- Antihistamines
- Anti-Parkinson agents
- Skeletal muscle relaxers
- Opiate agonists
- Alcohol

*Natural or alternative medications*
- Ginsing
- St. John's Wort
- Valerium
- Dehydroepiandrosterone (DHEA)
- Ephedra
- Vitamin C

**Medications associated with insomnia**
- Amphetamines
- Caffeine
- Nicotine

**Table 7.3** Effect of common medications on sleep.

| Medication | Effect on sleep |
|---|---|
| Aspirin and ibuprofen in healthy subjects | Disrupts sleep architecture<br>Increases sleep latency<br>Increases nonrapid eye movement (NREM) stage 2 sleep<br>Increases slow-wave sleep<br>Decreases sleep efficiency<br>(*Note:* When pain is present, these medications may improve sleep) |
| Opioids | Increases NREM stage 2 sleep<br>Decreases slow-wave restorative sleep<br>Worsens SRBD or may induce it (respiratory depression) |
| Methadone | Known to precipitate central sleep apnea |
| Tricyclic antidepressants | Increase total sleep time<br>Increase NREM stage 2 (a stage when bruxism increases)<br>Decrease arousals<br>Increase rapid eye movement (REM) latency<br>Decrease REM |
| Trazodone | Increases total sleep time<br>Decreases sleep latency<br>(*Note:* good long-term sleep aid) |
| Benzodiazepines | Decreases sleep latency<br>Increases NREM stages 1 and 2<br>Increases total sleep time<br>Decreases slow-wave restorative sleep<br>Decreases REM<br>Increases sedation |
| Antidepressants (selective serotonin reuptake inhibitor) | Increase wakefulness<br>Decrease total sleep time<br>Slightly increase NREM stage 1<br>Decrease REM<br>May induce insomnia<br>May cause sleep bruxism |

*Sources:* Adapted from (1) Lee-Chiong T. Sleep: A Comprehensive Handbook. Hoboken, NJ: John Wiley & Sons. 2006. (2) Kryger MH, Roth T, and Dement WC. Principles and Practice of Sleep Medicine. Philadelphia: Elsevier/Saunders. 2005. (3) Pagel JF. Medications effects on sleep. In: Attanasio R and Bailey DR, eds. Sleep Disorders: Dentistry's Role (Dental Clinics of North America, 45:4). Philadelphia: W.B. Saunders. 2001;855–865.

- Corticosteroids
- Theophyline

## Medications for the treatment of insomnia
- Sonata (zaleplon)
- Ambien (zolpidem)

- Lunesta (eszopiclone)
- Dalmane (flurazepam)
- Restoril (temazepam)
- ProSom (estazolam)
- Halcion (triazolam)—increases NREM stage 2 and interferes with slow-wave sleep
- Rozerem (ramelteon)—acts on melatonin receptors (M1 and M2)

## Medications that impact respiratory drive
*May have an effect on OSA and chronic obstructive pulmonary disease*
- Benzodiazepines
- Barbiturates
- Narcotics
- Topamax

*Antihypertensives' effects on sleep*
- Beta agonists (Propranolol)
    Increase wakefulness
    Increase NREM stage 1
    Decreased REM
- ACE inhibitors: Lotensin, Vasotec, Monopril, Zestril, Accupril, Altace
    Increased insomnia
- Diuretics (HCTZ)
    Drowsiness
- Calcium agonists
    No sleep study data

## Medications that increase slow-wave sleep
- Gabatril (tiagabine)
- Gabapentin (Neurontin)
- Pregabalin (Lyrica)
- Trazadone (Desyrel)
- Mirtazepine (Remeron)
- Valdoxan (Agomelatine)—a new antidepressant that is in the third phase of clinical trials; also increases slow-wave sleep

For further details, it is recommended that each specific medication be evaluated with the use of current literature dedicated to this topic.

When evaluating a patient who has a sleep disorder, medication use needs to be taken into consideration as a factor. One study demonstrated that the use of an antidepressant or antihypertensive increases the risk for OSA.[5] The use of these two agents at the same time increases the risk for OSA significantly.

## Temporomandibular disorders assessment

It is important to be aware of a patient's status relative to past or existing TMD, which may involve the temporomandibular joint (TMJ) and/or the masticatory muscles. Although the TMD evaluation is often included as part of the initial new patient examination for every patient in a dental practice, a number of patients that present with a TMD condition may also have an underlying sleep disorder, and this may affect the overall management plan of the patient.

If a TMD condition is present, it is important to document its existence so that it can be further assessed should an OA be fabricated for OSA and/or snoring at some point in the future. For example, if OA therapy is being considered for management of an intracapsular disorder, such as a recent onset of a disc displacement with reduction, and there is also an OSA condition, then an OA design can be considered that may address both issues.

### *Temporomandibular joint*

In addition to recording any findings regarding sounds and tenderness to palpation of the TMJs, there should be documentation regarding the patient's mandibular range of motion.

A screening assessment of the TMJs may include the following components:

- Previous treatment, including OA therapy
- Joint tenderness (capsule, retrodiscal)
- Joint sounds (clicking, crepitus, popping)
- Range of motion (opening, protrusion, lateral excursions)

### *Masticatory and cervical muscles*

Palpation of the muscles of the head and neck should be performed to determine if there is any local tenderness or referred pain patterns. An awareness of these masticatory and cervical muscles is essential in determining the source of pain. The muscles that were found to be tender should be recorded for future reference.

## Oral airway evaluation

The following components should comprise the oral airway evaluation:

- Uvula
    Normal
    Enlarged/swollen
    Elongated
    Surgically removed

- Soft palate
  Normal
  Enlarged/swollen
  Slopes downward into the oropharynx
- Gag reflex
  Normal
  Diminished
  Absent
  Exaggerated
- Tonsils grade (0, I, II, III, IV)

## Dentition and supporting structures

It is important that the patient's current dental health status be recorded, which includes the teeth as well as the supporting structures. The occlusion and maxillomandibular relationship are major factors because of the concern that exists for potential changes in these areas that may be associated with the use of an OA.

Components of documentation for the dental and supporting structures evaluation include the following:

- Classification of occlusion (I, II, III; Div 1, Div 2)
- Deep bite
- Crossbite
- Maxillary incisors (retroclined, normal)
- Wear facets on the teeth (mild, moderate, severe)
- Periodontal status (no disease, gingivitis, recession, halitosis, abfraction, teeth mobility)
- Hard palate (narrow, high)
- Lip seal (strained/forced, no lip seal, lips dry/chapped)

### Importance of lip seal

Assessment of the patient's ability to maintain a lip seal and identification of any indicators for mouth breathing are critical components of the oral airway evaluation. Lack of a lip seal and the resulting mouth breathing pattern or habit is also indicative of an individual who may have the following: (1) difficulty breathing comfortably through the nose, (2) allergies, or (3) nasal airway obstruction. Both mouth breathing and limited nose breathing may contribute to an increase in inspiratory pressure as well as to snoring and OSA because of airway compromise (Figure 7.2).

It is helpful to recognize someone who may be a mouth breather. When an individual is sitting comfortably in a relaxed position, the lips should be comfortably together without any appearance of being strained. If the lips are not in contact and are apart, this is usually indicative of a chronic mouth breathing pattern, often referred to as an obligate mouth breather. When this same individual attempts to close the lips, it will appear strained. In

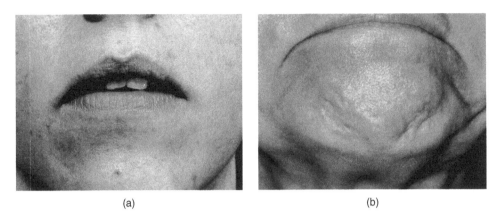

(a)                                                    (b)

**Figure 7.2**    Mouth breathing appearance: (a) lips apart at rest and (b) forced or strained lip seal.

addition, the chin may appear tight or wrinkled, oftentimes a sign of increased mentalis muscle activity (Figure 7.3).

## Tongue assessment

Evaluation of the tongue includes observation for scalloping, size, or coated surface. In addition, the Mallampati score assesses tongue position relative to the soft palate as well as visualization of the oropharynx as indicators of the risk for OSA. The assessment's scoring has been revised from

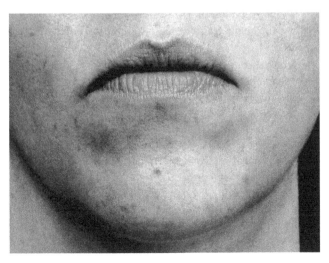

**Figure 7.3**    Lips closed at a relaxed position without strain—note the lack of wrinkling in the area of the chin.

when it was initially developed and used by anesthesiologists to assess the difficulty of intubation.[6]

To determine a score, the mouth is held open with the tongue at a rest position as compared to the version utilized by the anesthesiologist where the tongue is protruded. In both cases, the position is graded from I to IV (Figure 7.4).

As the degree of obstruction of the oropharyngeal airway and the soft palate increases, the risk for OSA also increases. It has recently been demonstrated that as the score progresses from I to IV, the potential severity of OSA also worsens.[7] The study also found that for each 1-point increase in the Mallampati score, the odds of having OSA were more than twice as likely, and the apnea–hypopnea index (AHI) may increase more than 5 events per hour (Table 7.4).

Evaluation of the tongue should include the following components:

- Large
- Coated
- Scalloped
- Fissured
- Tongue-tied (lingual frenum restricts movement)
- Mallampati score: o I o II o III o IV

### Uvula assessment

The appearance of the uvula may also indicate the risk for OSA and/or snoring. The uvula may appear enlarged, swollen, elongated, and even bruised (Figure 7.5). Negative intrapharyngeal pressure is associated with a narrowed or obstructed airway, and these clinical findings may be a result of the mechanical trauma associated with the snoring and obstructive breathing events.

### Soft palate assessment

Observation of the soft palate is another necessary component of the evaluation by the dentist because of the clinical significance of the slope or length of the soft palate. The more that the soft palate slopes down into the oropharyngeal space, the greater is the potential impact for airway obstruction. In addition, the more the soft palate slopes downward, the higher the Mallampati score.

As with the uvula, the soft palate may also appear swollen from the mechanical trauma associated with snoring and/or OSA.

### Gag reflex

In patients who snore or have sleep apnea, the gag reflex may be impacted by neurological alterations in this response, resulting in a less pronounced

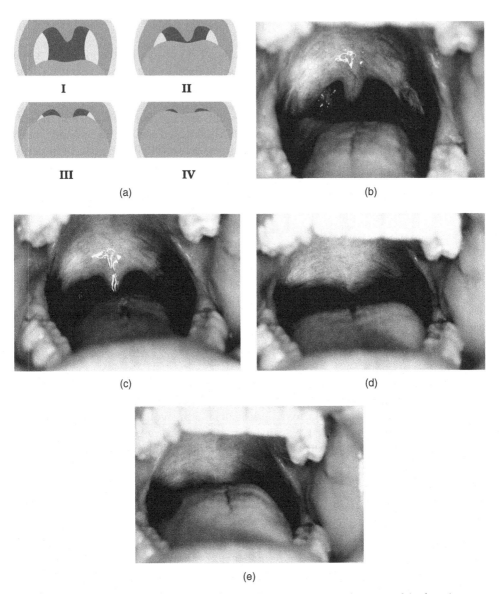

**Figure 7.4** Illustrations of the Mallampati score: (a) diagrams of the four designations (I—a clear view of oropharynx, uvula, and soft palate; II—a limited view of the orpharynx with a view of most of the uvula and soft palate; III—unable to view the oropahrynx, the uvula, and only a portion of the soft palate; IV—view of oropharynx, uvula, and soft palate totally obstructed by the tongue), (b) example of the Mallampati I, (c) example of Mallampati II, (d) example of Mallampati III, and (e) example of Malampati IV.

**Table 7.4**  Example of effect of Mallampati score on OSA and AHI.

| Mallampati score | Odds ratio for OSA | Possible AHI |
| --- | --- | --- |
| I | 1 | 5 |
| II | 2.5 | 10 or more |
| III | 5 | 15 or more |
| IV | 7.5 | 20 or more |

*Source:* Adapted from Nuckton TJ, Glidden DV, Browner WS, et al. Physical examination: Mallampati score as an independent predictor of obstructive sleep apnea. Sleep. 2006; 9(7):903–908.

or even absent reflex. Even though an altered gag reflex may not always be present, it is advisable to screen for this clinical finding. If this is suspected during the course of a routine oral examination, then the possibility of snoring and/or OSA should be considered.

### Tonsils assessment

The enlargement of the tonsils may contribute to airway obstruction as well as an increased tendency for mouth breathing. This enlargement may also compromise the airway and contribute to snoring and OSA. This is particularly true in children and adolescents. In adults, this may also be the case but to a lesser degree.

The standard grading system for the tonsils rates them on a scale from 0 to IV, with 0 indicating that the tonsils are absent and grade IV indicates they are grossly enlarged (Figure 7.6).[8]

Typically as one goes through puberty, the size of the tonsils will decrease to a grade I or 0. In some situations this will not occur, and this is when they may impact the airway. Thus, the evaluation of the tonsils should be a routine part of the oral airway evaluation.

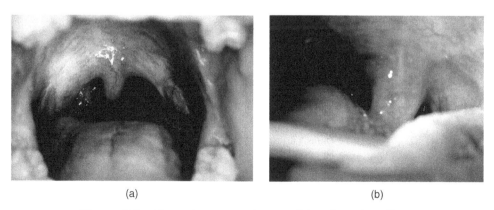

(a)                                             (b)

**Figure 7.5**  The uvula: (a) normal size and (b) enlarged/swollen.

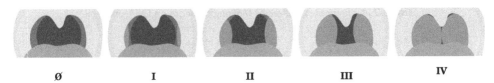

Ø          I          II          III          **IV**

**Figure 7.6**    Typical grading of the tonsils: 0, removed or not visible if present; I, barely visible; II, enlarged with limited obstruction; III, enlarged with significant obstruction; and IV, grossly enlarged and obstructive ("kissing tonsils").

## Nasal airway evaluation

Nose breathing is the preferred mode of respiration despite the fact that many patients are habitual mouth breathers. Chronic mouth breathing is often associated with nasal airway obstruction. It is within the scope of the dentist to perform a nasal airway screening to assess the status of the nasal airway.

To help determine if the patient perceives nasal airway problems during the last month, the use of a scale called the Nasal Obstruction Symptom Evaluation (NOSE) Instrument may be utilized (Figure 7.7).[9]

In addition to the instrument itself, a visual analog scale is used to assess the difficulty on average for nose breathing. The results may be helpful in

**Nasal Airway / Breathing Assessment**
Recently how much have the following
conditions been a concern or problem
(place a mark on the line that
best describes your situation)

Minimal    Mild    Moderate    Severe

Nasal
congestion    |———————————————————————|
stuffiness
obstruction

Difficult to
nose breathe    |———————————————————————|
when sleeping

Difficult to
nose breathe    |———————————————————————|
with exercise
or exertion

Difficult to
nose breathe    |———————————————————————|
in general

**Figure 7.7**    The nasal airway/breathing assessment. (From Stewart MG, Witsell DL, Smith TL, et al. Development and validation of the Nasal Obstruction Symptom Evaluation (NOSE) scale. Otolaryngol Head Neck Surg. 2004; 130:157–163.)

determining if further evaluation is needed or if a referral to an otolaryngologist may be indicated. The assessment may also be useful in evaluating if treatment designed to improve the nasal airway has been successful.

The nasal airway is important because it performs three main functions, basically acting as the carburetor of the body. Air passing through the nose is warmed and humidified to an 80% level, both of which contribute to the absorption of oxygen by the lungs.[10] In addition, air passing through the nose is also filtered.

## Nasal airway anatomy

The anatomy of the nasal airway starts at the outer portion of the nose with the alar rim or external nasal valve and the columella that separates the two nostrils (Figure 7.8).

Evaluation of the inner portion of the nose reveals structures that may act to restrict nasal airflow. To observe the inner anatomy of the nose, it is helpful to use a nasal speculum (Figure 7.9). This instrument allows for an improved visualization of the inferior turbinates, the nasal septum, and the nasal valve.

In order to adequately see inside the nose, a bright light source is necessary. This can be obtained with a bright flashlight or with a nasal illuminator (Figure 7.10). The internal aspect of the nose can then be better visualized to assess some critical structures.

The perceived nose is actually two separate components. The portion that is more anterior is the externally visible portion of the nose, and the

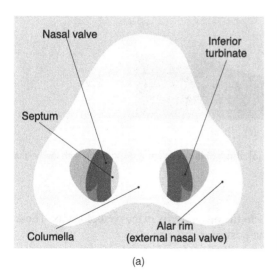

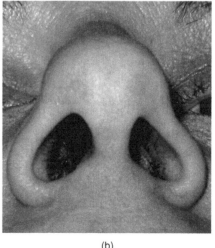

(a)                                                    (b)

**Figure 7.8**    The nose. It demonstrates the outside area of the nose—the part surrounding the nose is termed the alar rim and the mid-section that divides the two nostrils is termed the columella. (a) Diagram of nose and (b) clinical picture of nose.

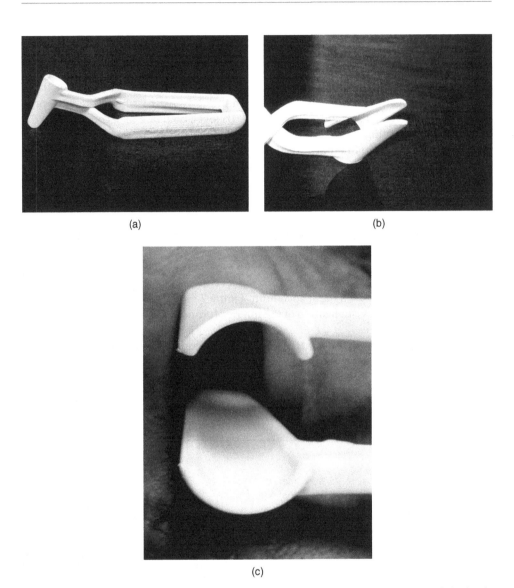

**Figure 7.9** Nasal speculum: (a) disposable speculum, (b) speculum with the beaks opened, and (c) speculum in use.

part behind this that connects to the oropharynx is the nasopharynx. These two areas are separated by the posterior choanae.

The use of a nasal speculum will allow for observation of the following structures (Figure 7.11):

- The turbinates, especially the inferior turbinates, are present at the lateral aspect of the nasal airway.

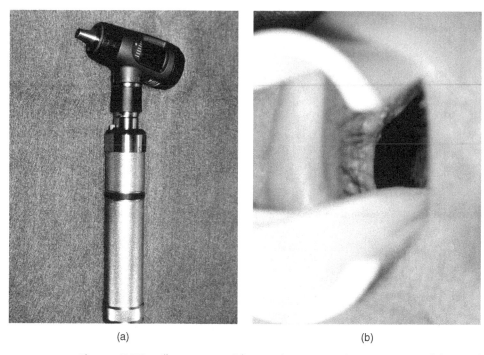

(a)                                         (b)

**Figure 7.10**   Illuminator used for visualization into the nose as part of the nasal airway evaluation: (a) otoscope with adaptor for visualization and (b) visualization of the inside of the nose with light source in use.

- The nasal septum is at the midline of the nose and separates it into two compartments. Deviation of the septum may be observed.
- The nasal valve can be assessed to determine its width and degree of opening. This is not an anatomic structure, but rather an area whose boundary is the nasal septum and the inferior turbinates.

It is the nasal valve that regulates airflow through the nose. This valve is subject to many different conditions that can affect it such as allergy, inflammation of the inferior turbinates, and nasal septum deviation. However, airflow can also be impacted by the presence of other pathology in the nose, such as polyps.

Even a small change in the opening of the nasal valve may result in significant improvement, and this observation is referred to as Poiseuille's Law. Regarding the nasal airway, the inspiratory pressure required to draw air through the nose is impacted by the fourth power of the radius. Thus, a small change or improvement in the opening of the nasal valve significantly decreases the pressure required to inspire air. An increase in nasal airway obstruction leads to an increase in inspiratory pressure, which results in airway collapse and an increased risk for OSA.[11]

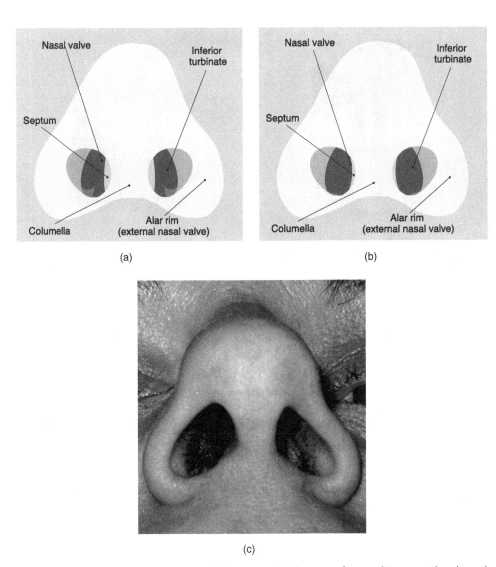

(a)

(b)

(c)

**Figure 7.11** View inside the nose: (a) diagram of nose, (b) nose with enlarged inferior turbinates and narrowed nasal valves, and (c) clinical picture of the nasal airway.

Components of the nasal airway evaluation should include the following:

- Nasal airway (open, obstructed, stuffy, septal deviation)
- Inferior turbinates, both right and left (normal, enlarged)
- Columella (normal width, wide, compression improves breathing)
- Nasal valve, both right and left (open/normal, narrow, blocked)
- Effect of nasal dilation (Cottle Test) (improved breathing; no effect)

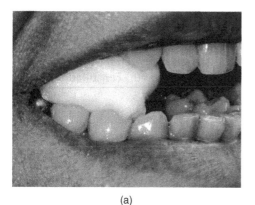
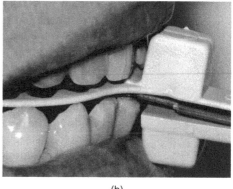

(a)                                                  (b)

**Figure 7.12**  Means of testing mandibular position to determine if there is sub-jective improvement in the airway and if the snoring is reduced or eliminated: (a) using cotton rolls between the posterior teeth and (b) using the George Gauge.

### Subjective airway testing

As a component of the overall SRBD evaluation, it is important to deter-mine if the patient experiences an improvement in their breathing and/or a reduction in the ability to snore if the mandible is repositioned. This test-ing may be assessed by using a prop, such as a bite stick, or by placing half of a cotton roll between the maxillary and mandibular posterior teeth to open the vertical between 2 and 5 mm, and subsequently having the patient move the mandible to an edge-to-edge position (Figure 7.12).

With this repositioning exercise, the patient needs to maintain a lip seal as well. With the mandible repositioned, have the patient practice breath-ing mainly through the nose. Determine at this point if they perceive an improvement in their breathing.

To assess if the mandibular repositioning has affected the ability to snore, ask the patient to make a snoring sound prior to the repositioning exercise. Subsequently with the mandible opened and advanced, have the patient attempt to snore. With the mandible opened and advanced, the abil-ity to snore is often decreased and/or eliminated.

If the airway does not feel as if it has improved or if the snoring was not significantly impacted, then additional attempts with this same exercise at varying degrees of opening and/or advancement may be attempted. The results of this type of testing can be documented on the screening evalua-tion form.

## MANAGEMENT PLAN

Once all the data from the various components of the evaluations have been completed, a plan of action needs to be presented to the patient. This management plan may take on a number of options depending on the scope of the treatment and the degree to which the practitioner wishes to be involved. The overall outcome most often will involve either the patient going on for further testing such as a sleep study or getting an OA. Regardless, various options should be explored as part of the consultation:

- Schedule
    Consultation with the dentist
    Schedule a more detailed evaluation
- Refer patient for a sleep study or to the physician
- Patient had a sleep study—obtain a copy for review
- Patient tried positive airway pressure therapy and/or had surgical intervention—consider OA therapy
- Schedule for OA therapy
- Need additional records
    Panoramic radiograph
    Cephalometric radiograph
    Cone beam imaging
    TMJ tomograms
- Refer for
    Physical therapy
    Myofunctional therapy
    Otolaryngology evaluation
- Recommend
    Commercial nasal dilator (e.g., Breathe Rite© strips)
    Commercial sinus rinse (e.g., Neil Med© Sinus Rinses)

## CONCLUSION

The evaluation of the patient presenting for dental care also should be viewed as an opportunity to screen for health-related issues as well, and SRBD is no exception. A particular case in point is the screening of the periodontally involved patient who is at risk for cardiovascular disease. There are similar findings that may indicate a risk for SRBD.

Once the possibility of SRBD is recognized, then additional steps can be taken to further evaluate the patient. The outcome may lead to the ability to provide a service, such as a management plan and even treatment (e.g., OA therapy) that can ultimately improve the patient's quality of sleep and hence their quality of life.

## REFERENCES

1. Schwarting S and Netzer NC. Sleep apnea screening for dentists—political means and practical performance. Abstract from annual meeting of the Associated Professional Sleep Societies, Salt Lake City, UT, June 17–22, 2006.

2. Bian H. Knowledge, opinions, and clinical experience of general practice dentists toward obstructive sleep apnea and oral appliances. Sleep Breath. 2004; 8(2):85–90.

3. Johns MW. A new method for measuring daytime sleepiness: the Epworth Sleepiness Scale. Sleep. 1991; 14(6):540–545.

4. McNicholas WT and Phillipson EA. Breathing Disorders in Sleep. Philadelphia: W.B. Saunders. 2002; 22.

5. Farney RJ, Lugo A, Jensen RL, et al. Simultaneous use of antidepressant and antihypertensive medications increase likelihood of diagnosis of obstructive sleep apnea. Chest. 2004; 125(4):1279–1285.

6. Friedman M, Tanyeri H, La Rosa M, et al. Clinical predictors of obstructive sleep apnea. Laryngoscope. 1999; 109:1901–1907.

7. Nuckton TJ, Glidden DV, Browner WS, et al. Physical examination: Mallampati score as an independent predictor of obstructive sleep apnea. Sleep. 2006; 9(7):903–908.

8. Fairbanks DNF, Mickelson SA, and Woodson BT. Snoring and Obstructive Sleep Apnea. 3rd ed. Philadelphia: Lippincott Williams & Wilkins. 2003.

9. Stewart MG, Witsell DL, Smith TL, et al. Development and validation of the Nasal Obstruction Symptom Evaluation (NOSE) Scale. Otolaryngol Head Neck Surg. 2004; 130:157–163.

10. Pevernagie DA, De Meyer MM, and Claeys S. Sleep, breathing and the nose. Sleep Med Rev. 2005; 9:437–451.

11. Friedman M, Tanyeri H, Lim JW, et al. Effect of improved nasal breathing on obstructive sleep apnea. Otolaryngol Head Neck Surg. 2000; 122:71–74.

12. Weiss TM, Atanasov S, and Calhoun KH. The association of tongue scalloping with obstructive sleep apnea and related sleep pathology. Otolaryngol Head Neck Surg. 2005; 133(6):966–971.

# Imaging for sleep-related breathing disorders

8

## CONCEPTUAL OVERVIEW

Imaging of the airway and related structures is used for a variety of reasons. For the most part, imaging has been utilized in an effort to measure anatomical structures of the airway, to understand the dynamics of the airway with and without therapeutic interventions, and to better understand the pathophysiology of sleep-related breathing disorders (SRBD).

In the dental management of SRBD, the use of imaging to predict whether an individual may be at risk for obstructive sleep apnea (OSA) or snoring is limited at this time. As techniques are developed and refined, the possible use of imaging may be of some benefit. Currently, imaging as it relates to the diagnosis of upper airway compromise as well as to assess the dynamics of airway collapse is mainly for research purposes.

## IMAGING IN THE DENTAL OFFICE FOR SRBD

The use of imaging associated with the treatment of SRBD in dentistry may be considered in three circumstances:

1.  To predict the presence or risk in an individual for SRBD
2.  To assess dental and related structures pertaining to the treatment of SRBD, primarily with an oral appliance (OA)
3.  To determine if mandibular repositioning will improve the airway

There are a number of imaging options for the dentist to consider related to these three circumstances (Table 8.1).

**Table 8.1** Imaging options related to sleep-related breathing disorders and mandibular repositioning.

| Condition | Imaging option |
|---|---|
| Predict SRBD | Cephlalometric X-ray |
| | Cone beam CT |
| | Pharyngometry |
| Assess condition of dental and related structures | Panoramic X-ray |
| | Cephalometric X-ray |
| | Cone beam CT |
| | Cone beam CT |
| Determine if mandibular repositioning will improve the airway | Pharyngometry |

The three most common imaging options that can be utilized are computed tomography (CT), magnetic resonance imaging (MRI), and nasal-pharyngoscopy. These modalities are used on a limited basis and typically are not employed in the treatment of SRBD.

## Computed tomography and magnetic resonance imaging

CT and MRI scans may be useful if other pathology is being investigated as a possible factor in patients with sleep disorders. These imaging modalities have been shown to be resourceful when a secondary medical or neurological cause for a sleep disorder was suspected.[1,2]

CT is frequently employed by the otolaryngologist to evaluate the nasal airway and the sinuses, particularly for discerning the presence of any airway compromise from craniofacial structures.

CT has also been utilized to do research regarding the airway. A study using dynamic CT determined the impact of an OA on the airway, in particular examining the effect of the OA as it advanced the mandible, also known as anterior or mandibular repositioning, from its habitual maxillomandibular relationship.[3] The results demonstrated that the OA appeared to have a greater impact on the lateral aspect of the airway in the retropalatal and retroglossal areas.

MRI has been used extensively to study the dynamics of the upper airway in a variety of circumstances (Figure 8.1).[4,5] This particular imaging modality is not practical, nor it is indicated in everyday clinical use on a routine basis. It needs to be utilized in specific circumstances mostly related to research endeavors. It would be infrequent for the dentist to order this imaging modality for clinical purposes because of the associated expense to the patient, the difficulty for patients to initiate and maintain sleep in the noisy scanner, and the potential exclusion of some patients with metallic implants or pacemakers.

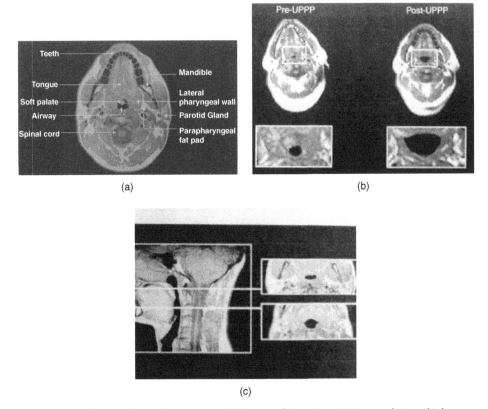

**Figure 8.1**    Cross-section MRI views of the airway: (a) general view, (b) the airway pre- and post-uvulopalatopharyngoplasty surgery, and (c) the airway at two levels: retropalatal and retroglossal. (Lee-Chiong T, ed. Sleep: A Comprehensive Handbook. Hoboken, NJ: John Wiley & Sons. 2006. Used with permission).

## Nasalpharyngoscopy (fiber optic pharyngoscopy)

Nasalpharyngoscopy, also known as fiber optic pharyngoscopy, is frequently used by the otolaryngologist to evaluate the airway. A flexible tube with a fiber optic light and camera allow for both dynamic and state-dependent visualization of the airway from the nose down to the larynx (Figure 8.2).

During this evaluation, the effect of inspiration with the nose and mouth closed, termed the Mueller maneuver, is observed.[6] This clinical technique replicates the effect of obstructive events in the airway, thereby indicating the impact of apnea events on the airway as well as identifying the specific site of obstruction associated with OSA. One study found that 60% of the sleep apnea patients had complete occlusion of the airway, 40% had multiple sites of obstruction, and there was reduced size along with increased collapsibility of the airway that correlated with an increase in the apnea–hypopnea index.[7]

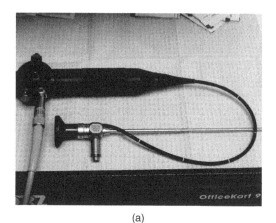

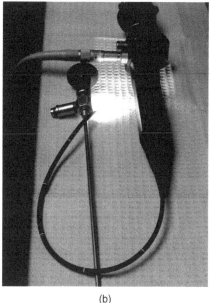

(a)                                                           (b)

**Figure 8.2**    View of rigid and flexible fiberoptic scope used to visualize the nasal airway and oropharynx down to the level of the epiglottis: (a) the rigid and flexible scopes and (b) the scopes showing the illumination.

## Pharyngometry

Pharyngometry, also known as acoustic reflection imaging (ARI), is another technique that has been utilized to evaluate the airway in patients with OSA and/or snoring (Figure 8.3). This modality emits a sound wave through the mouth that is helpful in the identification of the site(s) of narrowing from the oropharyngeal junction to the hypopharynx.

ARI may also determine the impact of mandibular repositioning on the airway and to what extent tongue space may increase. The technique for this modality is not standardized in terms of how it is performed, and it is therefore subject to the procedural handling by each individual user. The advantage of ARI is that it may assist the dentist in determining the potential for the success of OA therapy.[8] It was demonstrated that when the airway volume was increased as measured by ARI, there was a 60% chance that an OA would have a favorable prognosis. If the airway volume was unchanged, the possibility that an OA would not be of benefit was 95%. This modality may also be helpful with the postinsertion assessment of the OA relative to whether any further adjustments to the therapeutically induced maxillomandibular relationship may be helpful or necessary.

One study found that ARI could assist in predicting the risk for SRBD as related to gender and ethnic differences.[9]

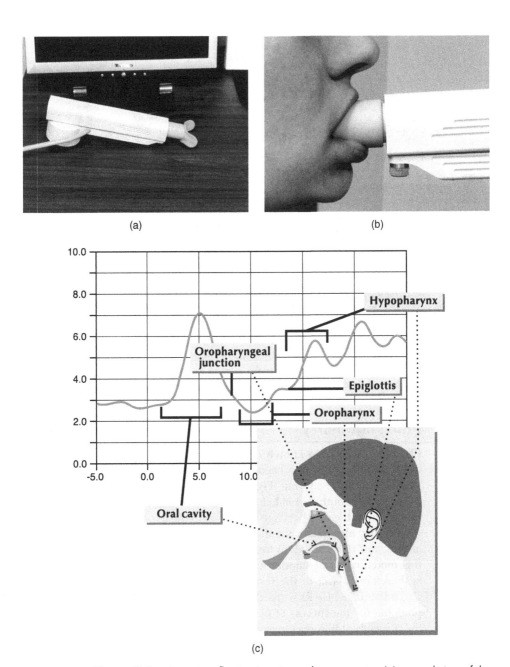

(a)

(b)

(c)

**Figure 8.3** Acoustic reflection imaging—pharyngometer: (a) general view of the wave tube that emits the sound waves and the oral mouthpiece—computer monitor can be seen in the background, (b) close-up view of the testing equipment in use, and (c) diagram of the image seen on the monitor that demonstrates the areas of the airway as they would viewed at the various levels of the airway.

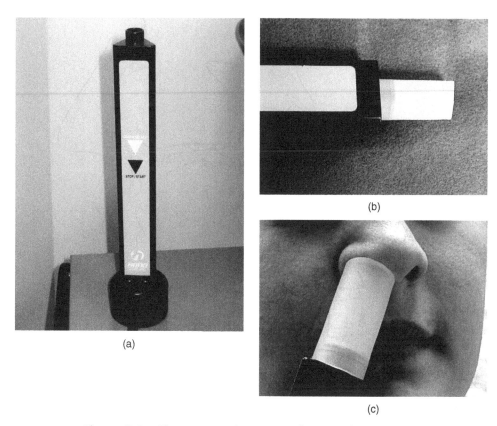

(a)

(b)

(c)

**Figure 8.4** Rhinometer used to acoustically image the nasal airway: (a) view of the rhinometer tube that emits the sound wave, (b) close-up view of the nasal interface used to emit the sound wave into the nasal airway, and (c) rhinometer in use—note the tight seal of the nasal interface.

This finding may have some possible impact in the future to use this device as a screening tool as well, but further evaluation and research are warranted.

A companion device, the rhinometer, may be utilized to evaluate the nasal area from the external nasal valve to the posterior choanae (Figure 8.4). This modality does not evaluate the nasopharynx; therefore, the area from the posterior choanae to the superior aspect of the soft palate is not analyzed. To do this, adjunctive imaging would need to be ordered as deemed necessary.

## Cephalometrics

Cephalometrics has been utilized for many years to assess a large number of craniomandibular osseous structures as well as to determine their impact on the airway as it relates to SRBD. The standards of practice on OAs

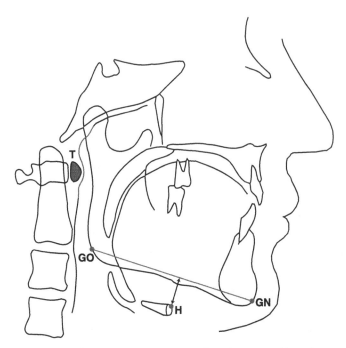

**Figure 8.5**   Cephalometric tracing to assess hyoid position. Note the perpendicular distance from the mandibular plane (Go-Gn) to the superior aspect of the hyoid (H). Note the anterior tubercle (T) of C-1 that is impacting the posterior aspect of the airway.

do not specifically recommend this imaging modality as part of the treatment, but the standards do indicate that cephalometrics can be used as an option if the clinician deems it necessary.[10]

At the current time, the use of cephalometrics seems to have a limited role. Historically, the airway has been visualized from an anteroposterior perspective to determine if it was compromised. However, this perspective was limited and it did not visualize the area in three dimensions.

In addition, a wide variety of classical cephalometric values have been reviewed to see if they can predict risk for SRBD. The one finding that has been repeatedly reliable as well as indicating a risk for a SRBD is hyoid position (Figure 8.5).[11,12] Outcomes demonstrated that the more inferior the hyoid was relative to the mandibular plane and the larger the distance between the hyoid and the mandible, the greater the risk for SRBD.

Another study also found that the lowered position of the hyoid bone was significant as a predictor of OSA independent of obesity.[13] In addition, the presence of a short mandibular corpus (body) was a relevant factor, and the study also demonstrated that a predisposition to OSA was associated with maxillary and mandibular retrognathism as well as a reduced facial height and deep bite.

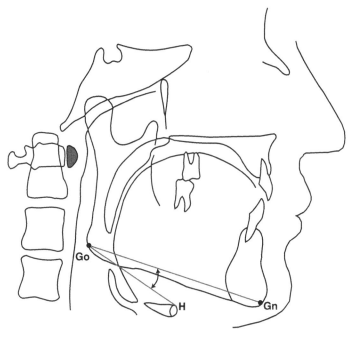

**Figure 8.6**  Cephalometric tracing to assess hyoid position. The angle from the mandibular plane (Go-Gn) to the superior aspect of the hyoid (H). As this angle increases, the hyoid moves down and posterior.

Another way of viewing this image is to look at the angle formed by the Go-Gn line to the hyoid (Figure 8.6). The greater this angle becomes, the lower and more inferior the hyoid is and hence the risk for OSA is increased.[14] This finding is relevant particularly to those who order cephalometric X-rays on a regular basis for orthodontic procedures.

The observation of the hyoid position needs to be observed because of its correlation as a potential risk factor for SRBD, and this finding alone should stimulate the need for further and more detailed investigation.

Another cephalometric method that can be used is to assess the position of the hyoid bone by simply using a line drawn from the most inferior-anterior point of the third cervical vertebrae to the point menton (Me) of the mandible (Figure 8.7). As such, the hyoid should be on the line or above it. If the hyoid is below this line, then it is considered that the risk for OSA increases.

A study also looked at the tubercle of the first cervical vertebrae.[11] There may be instances when this tubercle is protruded forward, thus creating a narrowing of the airway in the pharynx from the posterior aspect. The clinician may need to consider this possibility on the basis of the assessment of the patient's posture relative to the cervical spine.[15] As head posture

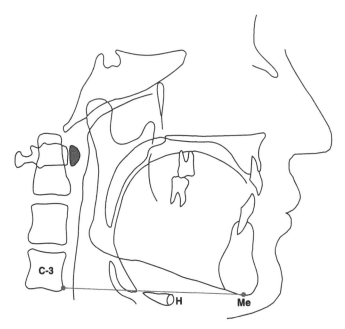

**Figure 8.7**  Cephalometric tracing to assess hyoid position, relative position of the hyoid (H), related to a line from menton (Me) to the inferior–anterior tip of the third cervical vertebrae (C-3).

changes, oftentimes in response to a compromised airway, the cervical spine is also impacted which may then impact the hyoid position.

Another possibility for compromise of the posterior pharyngeal wall may be the presence of osteophytes or small bony outgrowths associated with cervical spondylosis or a condition often termed ankylosing spondylosis (Figure 8.8).[16] This study demonstrated the impact of osteophytes on the compression of the posterior aspect of the pharyngeal wall and the improvement following their surgical removal. The presence of the osteophytes frequently may be associated with symptoms such as difficulty swallowing, throat pain, shoulder pain, and headaches.

A study assessing head shape as a predictor for snoring resulted in the development of the craniofacial risk index (CRI).[17] The CRI uses age, body mass index, and 14 cephalometric measurements as means of determining risk for snoring, and it was found to be effective 75% of the time.

## Cone beam computed tomography

Cone beam CT, also known as cone beam volumetric imaging (CBVI), is an imaging technology that has the potential to assess the airway along with the craniofacial structures in a three-dimensional perspective (Figure 8.9). A study that used CBVI to review the airway configuration in subjects with

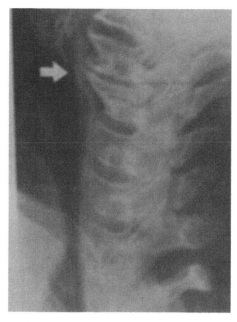

**Figure 8.8**    Osteophyte of the cervical spine and the impact on the airway from the posterior aspect.

OSA demonstrated the difference in airway volume and shape when comparing controls to individuals with OSA.[18] The ability to evaluate the airway volume as well as the anteroposterior dimension was found to be useful in discerning individuals at risk for SRBD.

Because this is new technology, the full scope of its possible use has not yet been determined. With what is known to date, cone beam imaging has been termed "virtual laryngoscopy," and a study indicated that a broad range of possibilities exists for this technology.[19] For example, it is feasible to employ the Mueller maneuver during CBVI because of the 9-second scan time.

Comparison of cone beam imaging to cephalometrics also demonstrated a moderate degree of variability in the assessment of the upper airway volume and area.[20] This finding could be used to plan the therapy,[21] and the cone beam modality may be a valuable tool in establishing or modifying mandibular position for OA therapy or in planning for surgical intervention.

## Panoramic radiograph

The panoramic radiograph should be utilized in the management of SRBD, especially if an OA is considered as part of the management plan (Figure 8.10). This imaging modality should be used to evaluate the dental

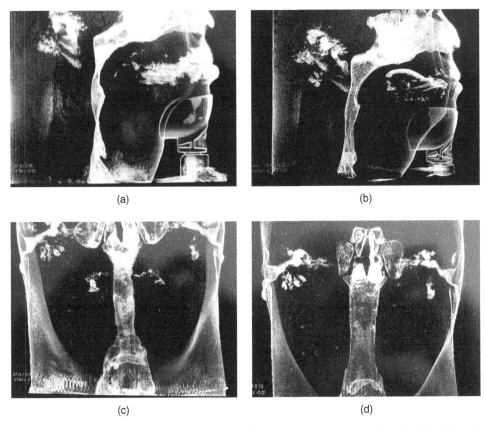

(a)  (b)

(c)  (d)

**Figure 8.9**  Cone beam images of a sleep apnea patient with and without the oral appliance in place; (a) and (b) are sagittal views and (c) and (d) are frontal views: (a) airway at normal jaw position, (b) airway with the mandible repositioned, (c) airway at normal jaw position, and (d) airway with the mandible repositioned.

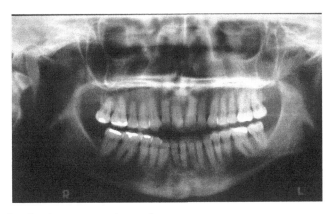

**Figure 8.10**  Panoramic radiograph.

structures of the patient and to look for any pathology that may be present. It can also be helpful to screen for any gross temporomandibular joint (TMJ) changes, to evaluate the nasal airway structures (e.g., turbinates and nasal septum), and to assess the sinuses.

## Tomography

Tomography, also known as tomograms, or other more advanced TMJ imaging modalities are not a standard of care for the SRBD patient, particularly if OA therapy is planned or being utilized. However, if temporomandibular disorder symptoms or signs are present, then additional more advanced and specific imaging may be indicated.[22] Tomography may be performed if condylar displacement or arthritic changes are of concern and more detailed osseous imaging is needed. In addition, MRIs can be performed if a soft tissue problem is of concern, particularly if a disc displacement within the TMJ is suspected.

Imaging is not needed to purely assess TMJ position when the mandible is being repositioned with an OA for dental management of SRBD. It has been demonstrated that mandibular repositioning OAs do not precipitate TMJ problems with long-term use.[23] In addition, there does not appear to be any alteration in TMJ function.

# CONCLUSION

The use of imaging relative to SRBD has the potential to aid in determining the risk for these disorders as well as to assist with the diagnosis and management, particularly with application to the use of an OA. However, imaging is not a replacement for sound clinical diagnosis, and it should be utilized as an adjunct in the diagnosis, treatment planning, and treatment progress.

In the future, the utilization of imaging will take on a more definitive role as additional research demonstrates the usefulness of the various technologies. Also, the cost effectiveness and the availability of conducting an imaging study may be of value to both the clinician and the patient as an aid to improved diagnosis and treatment outcome.

# REFERENCES

1. Nishino S and Kanbayashi T. Symptomatic narcolepsy, cataplexy and hypersomnia, and their implications in the hypothalamic hypocretin/orexin system. Sleep Med Rev. 2005; 9(4):269–310.
2. Marcus CL, Trescher WH, Halbower AC, et al. Secondary narcolepsy in children with brain tumors. Sleep. 2002; 25(4):435–439.

3. Kyung SH, Park Y, and Pae E. Obstructive sleep apnea patients with the oral appliance experience pharyngeal size and shape changes in three dimensions. Angle Orthod. 2004; 75:15–22.

4. Schwab RJ. Radiographic and endoscopic evaluation of the upper airway. In: Lee-Chiong T, ed. Sleep: A Comprehensive Handbook. Hokoken, NJ: John Wiley & Sons. 2006; 393.

5. Schwab RJ. Imaging for the snoring and sleep apnea patient. In: Attanasio R and Bailey DR, eds. Sleep Disorders: Dentistry's Role (Dental Clinics of North America, 45:4). Philadelphia: W.B. Saunders Inc. 2001; 759–796.

6. Ritter CT, Trudo FJ, Goldberg AN, et al. Quantitative evaluation of the upper airway during nasopharyngoscopy with the Muller maneuver. Laryngoscope. 1999; 109:954–963.

7. Ye J, Wang J, Yang Q, et al. Computer-assisted fiberoptic pharyngoscopy in obstructive sleep apnea syndrome. ORL J Otorhinolaryngol Relat Spec. 2007; 69(3):153–158.

8. Viviano JS. Acoustic reflection: review and clinical applications for sleep-disordered breathing. Sleep Breath. 2002; 6(3):129–149.

9. Monahan K, Kirchner L, and Redline S. Oropharyngeal dimensions in adults: effect of ethnicity, gender, and sleep apnea. J Clin Sleep Med. 2005; 1(3):257–263.

10. Kushid CA, Morgenthaler TI, Littner MR, et al. Practice parameters for the treatment of snoring and obstructive sleep apnea with oral appliances: an update for 2005. Sleep. 2006; 29(2):240–243.

11. Hoekema A, Hovinga B, Stegenga B, et al. Craniofacial morphology and obstructive sleep apnea: a cephalometric analysis. J Oral Rehabil. 2003; 30(7):690–696.

12. Kulnis R, Nelson S, Strohl K, et al. Cephalometric assessment of snoring and nonsnoring children. Chest. 2000; 118:596–603.

13. Riha RL, Brander P, Vennelle M, et al. A cephalometric comparison of patients with the sleep apnea/hypopnea syndrome and their siblings. Sleep. 2005; 28(3):315–320.

14. Finkelstein Y, Wexler D, Horowitz E, et al. Frontal and lateral cephalometry in patients with sleep-disordered breathing. Laryngoscope. 2001; 111:634–641.

15. Rocabato M. Biomechanical relationship of the cranial, cervical and hyoid regions. J Craniomandib Prac. 1983; 1(3):61–66.

16. Fuerderer S, Eysel-Gosepath K, Schroder U, et al. Retro-pharyngeal obstruction in the association with osteophytes of the cervical spine. J Bone Joint Surg. 2004; 86-B(6):837–840.

17. Hans MG, Nelson S, Pracharktam N, et al. Subgrouping persons with snoring and/or apnea by using anthropometric and cephalometric measures. Sleep Breath. 2001; 5(2):79–91.

18. Ogawa T, Enrisco R, Shintaku WH, et al. Evaluation of cross-section airway configuration of obstructive sleep apnea. Oral Surg Oral Med Oral Pathol Oral Radiol Endod. 2007; 103(1):102–108.

19. Osorio F, Perilla M, Doyle DJ, et al. Cone beam computed tomography: an innovative tool for airway assessment. Anesth Analg. 2008; 106:1803–1807.

20. Kau CH and Richmond S. Three-dimensional cone beam computerized tomography in orthodontics. J Orthod. 2005; 32(4):282–293.

21. Shi H, Scarfe WC, and Farman AG. Upper airway segmentation and dimensions estimation from cone-beam CT image datasets. Int J Comput Assist Radiol Surg. 2006; 1:177–186.

22. de Leeuw R. General assessment of the orofacial pain patient. In: de Leeuw R, ed. Orofacial Pain: Guidelines for Assessment, Diagnosis and Management. 4th ed. Hanover Park, IL: Quintessence Publishing. 2008; 38.

23. de Almeida FR, Bittencourt LR, de Almeida CIR, et al. Effects of mandibular posture on obstructive sleep apnea severity and the temporomandibular joint in patients fitted with an oral appliance. Sleep. 2002; 25:507–513.

# Section 3

## Management of the Sleep-Related Breathing Disorder Patient

# Positive airway pressure therapy for sleep-related breathing disorders

## CONCEPTUAL OVERVIEW

For patients with obstructive sleep apnea (OSA), snoring, or upper airway resistance syndrome (UARS), the primary type of therapy is positive airway pressure (PAP)[1-3] (Figure 9.1). However, a significant challenge to both patients and health care practitioners is compliance (acceptance/adherence) to PAP therapy.[4]

Upper airway patency is maintained by PAP through a mechanism involving the creation of a "pneumatic splint." The PAP device produces a pressurized airflow that is delivered to the patient via a mask interface. This airflow subsequently creates a positive distension of the upper airway as well as changes in lung volume.

There are three primary types of PAP modes: (1) continuous positive airway pressure (CPAP), (2) bilevel positive airway pressure (BiPAP), and (3) autoadjusting positive airway pressure (APAP). A fourth mode receiving some attention is the expiratory pressure relief mode (Flexible CPAP).

There is a significant amount of published literature about PAP therapy. The purpose of this chapter is to present an emphasis on PAP therapy as it relates to the adult population with SRBD, in particular OSA.

## INDICATIONS FOR PAP THERAPY

For SRBD that involve collapse of the oropharyngeal soft tissues or narrowing of the upper airway (Figures 9.2–9.4), such as what occurs with OSA,

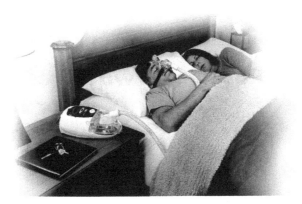

**Figure 9.1**    PAP is the primary type of therapy for OSA and SRBD. (© ResMed, 2008. Used with permission).

PAP is effective and accepted as appropriate therapy. There are published parameters for the use of PAP in the management of OSA.[1]

In essence, the objectives for managing OSA with PAP can include the following:[5–13] (1) reduction of excessive daytime sleepiness (EDS) that is related to other comorbid issues, such as motor vehicle accidents, cognitive

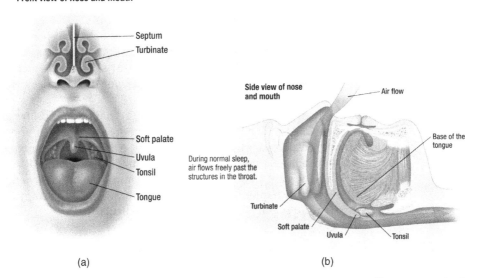

**Figure 9.2**    (a) Frontal view of normal oral and nasal airway. (© Krames Medical Publishing, 2009. Used with permission). (b) The normal upper airway allowing for an unobstructed pathway for breathing. (© Krames Medical Publishing, 2009. Used with permission).

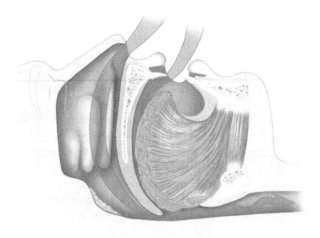

**Figure 9.3**   The partially obstructed upper airway that may result in snoring and/or hypopneic episodes. (© Krames Medical Publishing, 2009. Used with permission).

impairments, mood disorders; (2) prevention of cardiovascular sequela, such as high blood pressure; and (3) improvement of sleep for the bed partner, which usually involves the disturbing noises of snoring as well as the observation of apneic episodes.

PAP can be effective in obtaining these objectives and thereby improving the quality of life of individuals with OSA as well as the sleep of the bed partners.

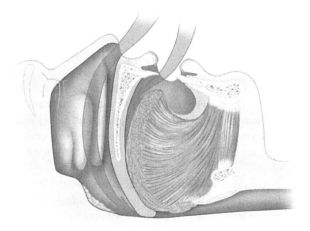

**Figure 9.4**   The completely obstructed upper airway that may result in apneic episodes. (© Krames Medical Publishing, 2009. Used with permission).

Besides effectiveness for management of moderate to severe OSA cases, PAP therapy may be effective for the management of mild OSA.[1] However, there is a greater propensity for those with mild OSA to demonstrate less adherence (compliance) to PAP therapy. It is important for even those individuals with mild OSA to know that there exists the increased risk for cardiovascular issues, such as hypertension (HT).[10–14]

The individuals with mild OSA or even primary (benign) snoring may not find appealing the alternative treatment options that include either surgical intervention of the upper airway tissues or the use of an OA. The remaining possible conservative options include weight loss, sleep positional changes, sleep hygiene modifications, or other alternative therapies.

As with other areas of medical care, there are Medicare guidelines for PAP therapy reimbursement, which can serve as references for the indications of PAP therapy.[15] If there is an apnea–hypopnea index (AHI) of 5–14 episodes/hour that represents mild OSA, then there must also be symptoms or signs of significant impairment. Impairments that qualify include EDS, HT, insomnia, mood disorders, and cardiovascular issues. These impairments are not required for individuals with an AHI of 15 or more episodes per hour that represent moderate to severe OSA.

The effectiveness of PAP therapy for each individual diagnosed with OSA is assessed during an attended polysomnogram (PSG) or sleep study. During the PSG visit, the type of PAP mask interface and the level of airflow pressure effective for managing the OSA are established. This determination may be done during a second sleep study, also known as a two-night study, or they may be performed during the latter portion of a single sleep study, also known as a split-night study.

## MECHANISMS OF ACTION

The flow of pressurized air from the PAP device most often travels through the nasal passages and upper airway, past the soft palatal tissues and tongue, and down the lower airway to the lungs. This pressurized airflow creates an airway patency in the area of the nasal valve as well as in the oropharyngeal area by a combination of anterior displacement of the tongue base and soft palatal tissue along with distension of the lateral pharyngeal walls. In essence, the PAP functions as a "pneumatic splint" (Figure 9.5) that precludes the upper airway from collapsing during sleep.[16,17]

Compared to atmospheric pressure, the intraluminal pressure from the PAP is positive, which results in a dilation of the upper airway. This increase in the cross-sectional area and volume of the upper airway has been demonstrated with computed axial tomography scanning as well as with magnetic resonance images (Figures 9.6 and 9.7).[18–20] Subsequent to the opening of the airway by the "pneumatic splint," there is a reduction of the upper airway muscle activity,[21,22] thereby lowering muscle resistance.

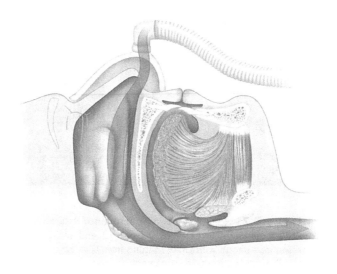

A mask over the nose gently directs air into
the throat to keep the airway open.

**Figure 9.5** The effectiveness of PAP in preventing collapse of the upper airway, also referred to as a "pneumatic splint." (© Krames Medical Publishing, 2009. Used with permission).

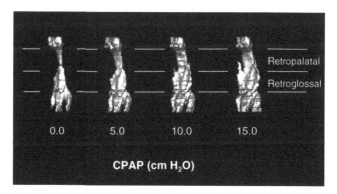

**Figure 9.6** Three-dimensional surface renderings of the upper airway in a normal subject demonstrating increased upper airway volume in the retropalatal and retroglossal regions with progressively greater CPAP (0–15 cm $H_2O$). (Schwab R. Imaging for the snoring and sleep apnea patient. In: Attanasio R and Bailey D, eds. Sleep Disorders: Dentistry's Role (Dental Clinics of North America; 45:4). Philadelphia: W.B. Saunders. 2001; 784. Reprinted with permission.)

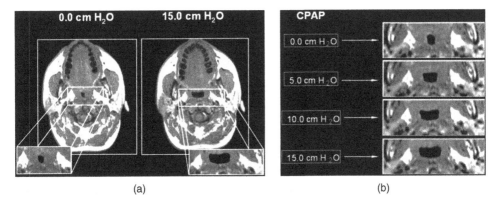

**Figure 9.7**    (a) Axial magnetic resonance image of the retropalatal region in a normal subject with CPAP of 0 cm $H_2O$ and of 15 cm $H_2O$. (b) Axial magnetic resonance image with CPAP ranging from 0 to 15 cm $H_2O$. Progressive increases in CPAP result in airway enlargement. (Schwab R. Imaging for the snoring and sleep apnea patient. In: Attanasio R and Bailey D, eds. Sleep Disorders: Dentistry's Role (Dental Clinics of North America; 45:4). Philadelphia: W.B. Saunders. 2001; 785. Reprinted with permission.)

# PATIENT COMPLIANCE (ACCEPTANCE/ADHERENCE)

Patient compliance, also referred to as acceptance and adherence, of PAP therapy is regarded as willingness of the patient to use the PAP device at home for at least 1 week.[4] Compliance is regarded as the patient using PAP therapy for more than 4 hours per night for more than 70% of the days.[23,24]

Through the use of memory cards, modems, or wire transfer of data from the PAP device to a computer, there can be an assessment of patient compliance (Figures 9.8 and 9.9). It is important to obtain adherence data early after the onset of PAP therapy since PAP users who are adherent during the initial 1–3 months are more inclined to continue with PAP therapy.[25,26]

However, in those individuals initially using PAP therapy, nonacceptance can vary from 5 to 50%, and by 3 years, an additional 12–25% no longer continue with PAP therapy.[4,27,28] When an aggressive systematic follow-up program for PAP treatment is employed that includes appropriate mask interface selection and fitting, heated humidification, patient education, objective assessment of adherence, and early intervention for adverse side effects, PAP user compliance can significantly increase with results varying from 40 to 80%.[23,29–34] These statistics are similar to adherence outcomes for chronic diseases managed by oral medications.

A poor fit of the mask interface, nasal symptoms (e.g., dryness, congestion, sore throat), and insufficient support from homecare providers

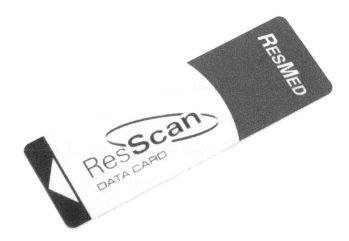

**Figure 9.8** An example of a data memory card for a PAP unit (© ResMed, 2008. Used with permission).

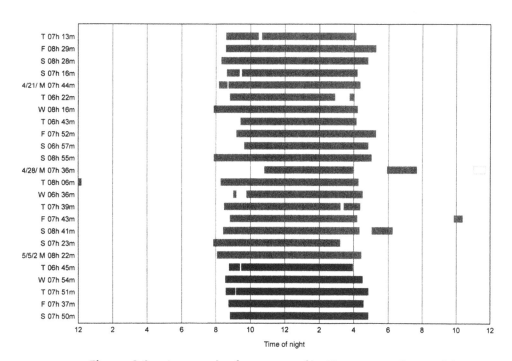

**Figure 9.9** An example of a usage profile. The printout reflects nightly usage relative to start and stop times. (© ResMed, 2008. Used with permission).

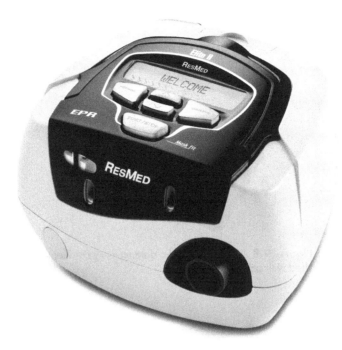

**Figure 9.10**    An example of a PAP device without a humidifier (ResMed S8 Elite) (© ResMed, 2008. Used with permission).

(e.g., follow-up) are typically the most common contributory factors to non-adherence to PAP therapy.[35]

## TYPES OF PAP MODES

Although CPAP has been used since its inception in 1981, there have been technological advancements resulting in other delivery modes for PAP: BiPAP,[36] APAP,[37–39] and, most recently, Flexible CPAP (Figures 9.10 and 9.11).[40]

### CPAP

The use of CPAP for the treatment of adults with OSA was first described in the literature in 1981.[41]

CPAP mode devices maintain a fixed or constant flow rate of air pressure during both inspiration and expiration. Through management that includes appropriate mask interface and possible use of airway humidification, many individuals find CPAP devices to be compatible for obtaining good sleep hygiene. Humidification can either be heated or at ambient

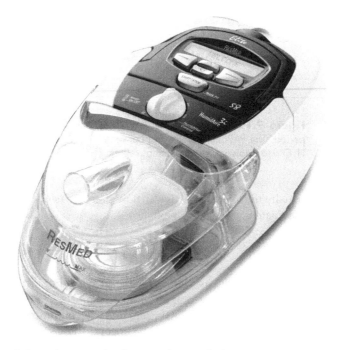

**Figure 9.11**    An example of a PAP device which incorporates a built-in heated humidifier (ResMed S8 Elite with H3i) (© ResMed, 2008. Used with permission).

room temperature, although PAP users typically prefer heated. CPAP devices are usually less expensive when compared to the other PAP modes.

## APAP

APAP mode devices employ a sensor-based mechanism that automatically adjusts the flow rate of air pressure by continually monitoring the upper airway patency.[37,38] Depending on the particular device, one or more respiratory factors are assessed, such as airflow limitations and impedence, which result in an air pressure that is constant during a respiratory cycle but variable during the course of a sleep period.[42–45] Adherence of PAP therapy may be improved because of the allowance of a variable mean pressure during the sleep period (Figure 9.12).

Although the built-in algorithms will differ per manufacturer, the common objective is to analyze airflow and provide feedback to the device to allow for a pressure change. So as not to cause a waking arousal, these changes in airflow pressure are made on a gradual basis. The lowest and highest pressure limits of the device are formatted by the health care practitioner. The APAP device can then provide the pressure as needed per the varying respiratory requirements during the sleep period, which is

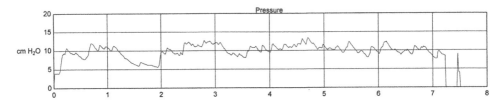

**Figure 9.12**    An example of PAP versus time for APAP treatment during a sleep period. The PAP unit autotitrated between a preset upper pressure limit of 20.0 cm $H_2O$ and a lower pressure limit of 4.0 cm $H_2O$.

usually the lowest effective airflow pressure needed to maintain upper airway patency.

## BiPAP

BiPAP mode devices allow for the provision of airflow pressures that reflect an inspiratory pressure higher than the expiratory pressure (Figure 9.13). Because some CPAP users find the continuous pressure during both inspiration and expiration to be uncomfortable, particularly the expiratory pressure, the BiPAP device's lower pressure during expiration can make

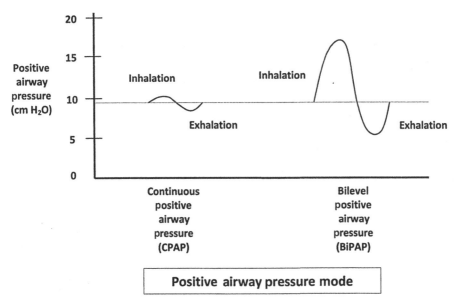

**Figure 9.13**    A comparison of inhalation and exhalation between CPAP and BiPAP regarding PAP. CPAP maintains a relatively steady positive pressure for both inhalation and exhalation. BiPAP provides a higher inhalation pressure and a lower exhalation pressure.

the device more tolerable to the user. A BiPAP device may lend to greater adherence for individuals who experience either aerophagia (i.e., forced ingestion of air into the stomach) or a reduced ventilatory drive.[46]

## Flexible CPAP

A recent technological advancement to further improve PAP therapy adherence has provided a CPAP variant that allows for a Flexible CPAP. By allowing the airflow pressure to go below the prescribed therapeutic airflow pressure in early expiration followed by a return of airflow pressure to the prescribed amount at the end of expiration, the Flexible CPAP mode can offer improved patient tolerance.

The C-Flex (Respironics, Murrysville, PA) is one model of this mode, and it allows for an alternating airflow pressure between inspiration and expiration on a breath-by-breath basis. During expiration, the device's airflow pressure decreases in proportion to the individual's expiratory airflow. By the end of the individual's respiratory expiration, the C-Flex's airflow pressure returns to the prescribed level of PAP.

A study demonstrated that adherence with the C-Flex was higher than with the traditional CPAP, although there were no significant differences between the two groups relative to subjective sleepiness or functional assessments.[40] Another study found no significant difference between the two groups relative to adherence and also found no significant differences relative to EDS and functional outcomes.[47]

# TYPES OF PAP MASK INTERFACES

Not only are the airflow pressure level and mode inherent to successful adherence with PAP therapy, but so is the challenge of selecting the optimal mask interface between the patient and the device. Mask interface issues can include discomfort from pressure of the mask against the nose or other facial areas, air leaks that can create noise or cause irritation of the eyes, and positional shifts of the mask that result from positional changes of the body during sleep.

As such, the development of various types of PAP mask interfaces by manufacturers has been robust. In addition, each type of mask interface is available in various sizes, typically small, medium, and large. Because the initial several weeks of PAP therapy are critical in establishing patient adherence, the American Academy of Sleep Medicine has recommended close follow-up evaluations to assess and manage issues arising from the PAP mask and/or device.[2]

Types of PAP mask interfaces (Figures 9.14–9.19) include the following: nasal mask, nasal pillows, full-face mask, oral-nasal mask, and oral mask. All PAP mask interfaces employ a varying type of headgear to maintain mask position. Sometimes it is necessary to also utilize a chin strap to

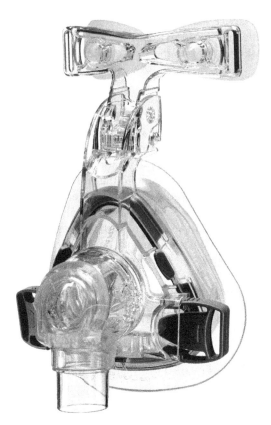

**Figure 9.14**    An example of a PAP nasal mask interface (ResMed Mirage Activa).
(© ResMed, 2008. Used with permission.)

prevent opening of the mouth for those individuals who mouth breathe during sleep.

To obtain an optimal seal, there are typically two types of material utilized for the actual area of the mask that interfaces with the patient's face. One is a thin, flexible plastic sleeve that inflates from the airflow pressure and thus presses an "air cushion" against the contours of the face, and another is a soft, gel-type material that adapts to the contours of the face.

One of the more challenging areas to obtain a seal is the bridge of the nose. When there are air leaks in this area, it is common for there to be a subsequent irritation of one or both eyes.[48]

The most common and traditional type of PAP mask interface is the nasal mask that fits over the entire nose, thereby creating a seal against the area above the upper lip but below the nares, against the cheek areas, and against the bridge of the nose.[49–51] For most PAP device users, opening of the mouth with subsequent mouth leaks is not an issue. The soft palatal tissues are pressed anteriorly against the posterior aspect of the tongue as a result of the positive airflow pressure in the nasopharynx.

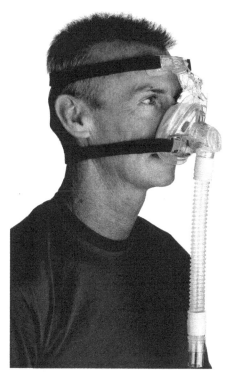

**Figure 9.15**   An example of a PAP nasal mask interface being worn (ResMed Mirage Activa). (© ResMed, 2008. Used with permission.)

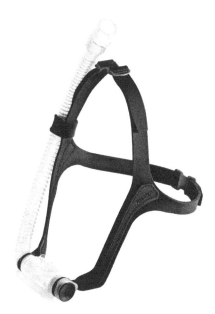

**Figure 9.16**   An example of a PAP nasal pillow interface system that utilizes interchangeable tube positions. (ResMed Swift II). (© ResMed, 2008. Used with permission.)

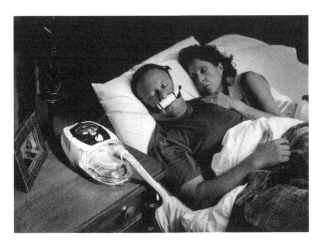

**Figure 9.17**   An example of a PAP nasal pillow interface system being worn (ResMed Swift II). (© ResMed, 2008. Used with permission.)

If a chin strap is not successful in maintaining mouth closure, if it is uncomfortable for the PAP user, or if there is an air leak causing eye irritation or a disturbing noise, then one of the other types of mask interfaces can be employed.

Another common type of PAP mask is the nasal pillows interface, which is composed of small nipple-type flexible rubber components that fit into

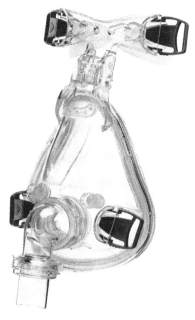

**Figure 9.18**   An example of a PAP full face mask interface. (ResMed UltraMirage Full Face). (© ResMed, 2008. Used with permission.)

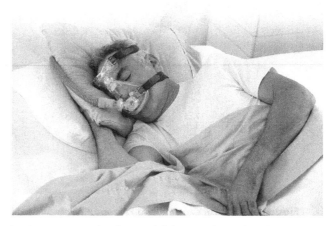

**Figure 9.19**    An example of a PAP full face mask interface being worn. (ResMed UltraMirage Full Face). (© ResMed, 2008. Used with permission.)

the nares (Figures 9.20 and 9.21). The position of the pillows is maintained by a small plastic holder connected to a head strap similar to the one used for the nasal mask. The pillows are inflated with the PAP device's airflow pressure, thus creating a seal against the nares. As with the nasal mask, some users may need to also employ a chin strap if they are mouth breathers.

Persistent mouth breathers for whom the chin strap is unsuccessful may find the oral-nasal, full-face, or the oral device interfaces helpful. Not having a patent nasal airway (e.g., nasal congestion) may be another reason for considering the use of such type of mask interface alternatives.

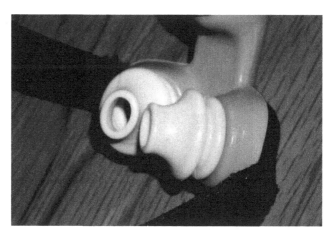

**Figure 9.20**    An example of a PAP nasal pillow interface system with soft flexible pillows.

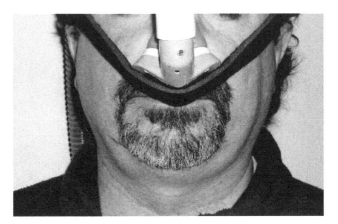

**Figure 9.21**    An example of a PAP nasal pillow interface system with soft flexible pillows being worn.

An oral-nasal mask or a full-face mask may be an appropriate alternative.[52–54] Airflow pressure to the nasal and oral airways is applied simultaneously with the use of an oral-nasal mask. For patients with mouth air leaks and drying of the tissues in the upper airway, a full-face mask interface can be effective, although it can be challenging to obtain a good mask fit around all borders. With both these types of interfaces, there are valves or orifices built-in to the mask component that provides the ability for inspiration of ambient air in the circumstance of losing airflow pressure from a power source failure of the PAP device.

The availability of the oral mask interface allows the opportunity to bypass the nose completely (Figure 9.22).[55] Because of the airflow pressure

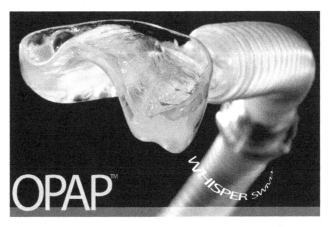

**Figure 9.22**    An example of a PAP oral appliance interface. (© OPAP—Aleksey Kozlov, 2009. Used with permission.)

against solely the oral tissues, it is usually necessary to provide heated humidification to minimize drying of those tissues. The oral mask can be uncomfortable to the user by virtue of its bulky design that incorporates flange components that fit behind and in front of the user's lips. Just as with the various nasal-involved type of masks, there can also be air leakage around the borders of the oral mask.

Most PAP devices employ the option to turn on a "mask-off" alarm that alerts the user of a significant air leak, which can occur from dislodgement of the mask interface from an adequate seal to the skin surface. Typically, the alarm awakens the PAP user and/or bed partner, and a simple readjusting of the mask interface resolves the leak and the alarm automatically ceases.

Each of the PAP mask interfaces needs the ability to clear out the user's exhaled $CO_2$. This is usually accomplished with the placement of a slit or orifice outlet either on the mask itself or at the junction of the mask and the hose that connects to the PAP device. This type of $CO_2$ outlet creates a necessary intentional leak.

From the aforementioned, it is obvious that mask fitting and comfort are critical factors and essential to enhanced patient adherence to PAP therapy. Typically, the prescribing sleep physician delegates this responsibility to either the respiratory therapist at the durable medical equipment company that will be providing the PAP device or the sleep technologist at the sleep laboratory that may provide the PAP unit.

# DETERMINATION OF PAP PRESSURE LEVELS

At either the split-night or two-night sleep study attended by the sleep technologist, the mask interface type is selected, and it then becomes necessary to establish the therapeutic level of airflow pressure from the PAP device.[1,56] This determination of effective PAP level is called PAP titration.

During the PAP titration portion of the sleep study, the sleep technologist typically uses remote control to incrementally increase the airflow pressure to determine levels when there is resolution of respiratory events, such as apneas, hypopneas, snoring, oxygen desaturations, and respiratory effort-related arousals. The effective PAP titration should normalize airway flow in the supine position as well as in rapid eye movement sleep. Protocols for PAP titration have been established.[57]

The attended PSG, or sleep study, provides an opportunity for a sleep technologist to account for patient discomfort, mask air leaks, mask position shifts, changes in body positions, stages of sleep, and other technical aspects such as the loss of PSG leads.[29,57–60] For example, it has been demonstrated that the therapeutic PAP pressure level was significantly higher in the supine position than in the lateral position in most individuals who were diagnosed with OSA.[60] Also, a study found that the therapeutic PAP pressure level was decreased with elevation of the bed's head portion,[59] and another study demonstrated that weight loss also allowed for a decrease of airflow pressure.[61]

The sleep physician subsequently reviews the recorded results of the PAP titration portion of the sleep study compared to the results from the non-PAP baseline portion of the sleep study. A therapeutic level of PAP is established and prescribed, and the patient is provided with a PAP device programmed to that therapeutic level of pressurized air. Pressure levels for effective PAP therapy can vary, but they are typically between 4 and 20 cm $H_2O$.

## BENEFITS OF PAP

Successful PAP therapy for the management of OSA can result in physical benefits for the user. It is well documented that PAP therapy will improve both EDS and quality of life.[3,62–67] In fact, one study found that some subjects diagnosed with OSA demonstrated improvements in EDS following only one sleep period of PAP therapy.[68]

By precluding apneic and hyponeic events, PAP therapy has been shown to be of benefit in reducing blood pressure in hypertensive patients who have sleep apnea,[69] decreasing nocturnal blood pressures,[70–72] and reducing diurnal blood pressures.[11,12] Also demonstrated in studies has been the improvement of neuropsychologic functioning with PAP therapy even in individuals diagnosed with mild OSA.[73,74]

As such, sleep quality is improved through the use of PAP therapy. Individuals diagnosed with sleep-disordered breathing who were users of PAP on a consistent basis showed improvement in EDS, motor vehicle accidents, memory loss, concentration deficiencies, mood disorders, and cognitive function outcomes.[75–77]

## ADVERSE SIDE EFFECTS OF PAP

There are adverse side effects associated with PAP therapy, and, if not addressed, these adverse side effects will decrease acceptance and adherence of PAP therapy.[78]

Adverse side effects of PAP therapy are common. A listing of the most common include dry nasal passages, rhinorrhea, and congestion, all of which can affect from 25 to 65% of PAP users.[79] These particular PAP users often also have had nasal symptoms prior to the use of PAP therapy. Other user complaints can include claustrophobia, irritation of the eyes, difficulty breathing the pressurized airflow, sore skin areas over the bridge of the nose (Figures 9.23 and 9.24) or the upper lip related to the mask interface, and even noise generated by the PAP device.

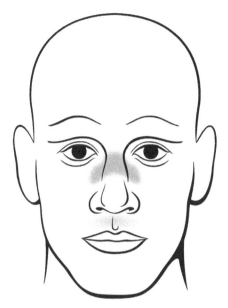

**Figure 9.23** Common pressure areas of mask interface systems that may result in skin irritation on the bridge of the nose and upper lip areas. (© ResMed, 2008. Used with permission.)

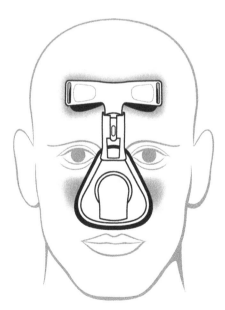

**Figure 9.24** Areas of resistance built into some mask interface systems, thus reducing pressure on sensitive areas. (ResMed Mirage system). (© ResMed, 2008. Used with permission.)

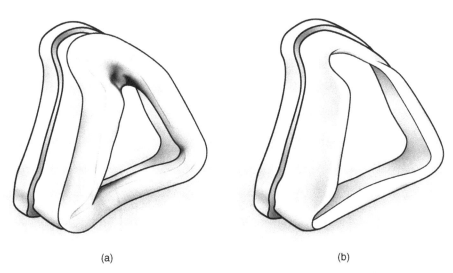

(a)                                                          (b)

**Figure 9.25**    An example of a dual-wall cushion technology designed to provide support and stability for a wide fit range and additional dispersion of weight and pressure, limiting contact of the cushion with the most sensitive areas of the face. (a) Outer lining of the dual-wall cushion and (b) inner lining of the dual-wall cushion. (ResMed Mirage system). (© ResMed, 2008. Used with permission.)

Many of the adverse side effects are mask interface related.[80] Despite the ability that PAP devices can take into account for air leaks at the mask interface (Figures 9.25–9.27), significant leaks that can occur with mouth opening may preclude the PAP device from producing ample airflow pressure to maintain airway patency.[81] The end results of these large

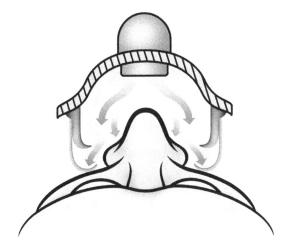

**Figure 9.26**    Cutaway shows how air pressure flows into the outer cushion of a dual-wall mask interface to enhance the seal, thus reducing the need for excessive head strap tension. (ResMed Mirage system). (© ResMed, 2008. Used with permission.)

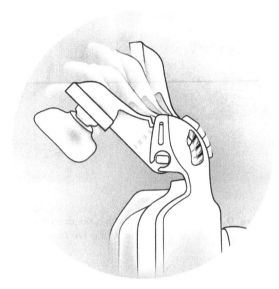

**Figure 9.27**    An example of an adjustable forehead support portion of a mask interface system that reduces pressure on a common sensitive area of the skin. (ResMed Mirage system). (© ResMed, 2008. Used with permission.)

air leaks can include dryness of the air passages as well as waking arousals, thereby counteracting the effectiveness of PAP therapy in managing OSA.

Sleep position of the head against a pillow while wearing a PAP mask may lend to discomfort from the pressure of the pillow against the mask or it may also lend to air leak from dislodgement of the mask by the pillow. Use of a specialized pillow, such as the PAPillow©, allows for the designed contours of the pillow's edge to allow the mask to extend beyond without pressure interference (Figure 9.28).

Nasal congestion is also common, and heated humidification of the PAP device's airflow may improve this situation. At times, it may be necessary to also treat the congestion with nasal steroid spray, nondrowsy antihistamines, or decongestants that the individual can use prior to sleep. A full-face mask or oral mask may also be considered,[52–54] but another alternative is surgical treatment if a nasal obstruction, such as a narrow nasal passage, can be identified as a contributing factor.[55,82]

Sometimes a PAP user will complain of difficulty breathing with the device's airflow pressure levels, but this is usually more common with CPAP than with BiPAP, APAP, or Flexible CPAP devices. Also, all that may be necessary is an adaptation period for the user to start the sleep period with an airflow pressure that is lower than the therapeutic level, and then the programmed PAP unit gradually increases the pressure over time as the patient accommodates. This is typically referred to as "ramp time."

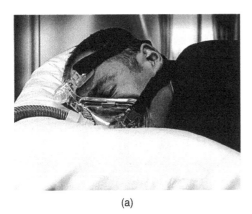
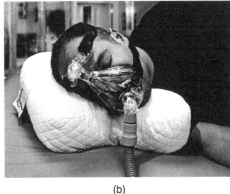

(a)                                          (b)

**Figure 9.28**    (a) CPAP user with a standard bed pillow. (© PAPillow, 2009. Used with permission). (b) CPAP user with a PAPillow. (© PAPillow, 2009. Used with permission.)

Noise complaints used to be more common with the older PAP devices. Most contemporary devices are significantly quieter. The noise that generally bothers either the PAP user or the bed partner is the sound created by the intentional leak of the PAP mask component as air is emitted from the orifice located in the mask or at the junction of the mask and the air tube that connects to the PAP unit. However, typically the bed partner will prefer such device-generated noise than the noise generated from the individual's snoring.

## OTHER CONSIDERATIONS

### Humidification

PAP devices can be fitted with either a cold passover (ambient temperature) humidifier or a heated humidifier. The initial PAP devices only had the cold passover humidification as an option. Subsequent generations of PAP devices incorporated heated humidification that could deliver more moisture than the cold passover version.

Since the mucosa of the nasal airway can dry and become tender from the passage of cold air, resistance in the nasal airway can increase without the use of any humidification. Studies have demonstrated that this nasal airway resistance caused by PAP therapy without humidification can result in significant air leak at the mask interface area from mouth opening, which in turn may cause further nasal airway resistance.[35,83] This may result in a cycle of nasal airway resistance, mask interface leaking, mouth breathing, increased nasal airway resistance, and worsening of the OSA. As a result of the decreased efficacy of the PAP therapy and decrease in patient comfort, PAP user compliance may be reduced.

With cold (passive) humidification, the PAP device generates air pressure that subsequently passes through a container that is partially filled with water. This mechanism allows for the air to absorb moisture as it passes over the surface area of the water in the container.

Heated humidification employs the use of a hot plate in the container of water, and the PAP device typically allows the user to modify the amount of heated humidification through a temperature control. As a result, the pressurized air has the advantage of being both warm and humid.

For the most part, PAP users tend to agree that heated humidification is more comforting to the nasal passages than is cold (passive) humidification. Both cold passover and heated humidification modalities result in greater PAP user satisfaction relative to no humidity. However, there were less adverse side effects with heated humidification when compared to cold passover humidification.[29,30]

Because an increase in infectious complications may be associated with PAP humidification,[84] it is recommended that the PAP user clean all the components involved (i.e., humidifier, hose, and mask) on a regular basis per the manufacturer's instructions.

## Ramp

Most PAP devices offer an optional "ramp" feature that allows the PAP user the opportunity to set a "ramp time," which is a period of gradual increase in airflow pressure from a low starting level to eventually reaching the prescribed therapeutic level. This period of time allows the patient to fall asleep when the airflow pressure is lower, thereby increasing the acclimation and comfort, and thus the successful adherence to PAP therapy.

## Traveling with CPAP

PAP devices need to be protected from damage during travel. PAP users who derive benefits from their PAP device should carry their devices in a carry-on bag, whether in automobile transit or air travel. Most airport security screening personnel are familiar with PAP devices, and they are allowed as a carry-on item. Nonetheless, it is recommended that the PAP user still obtain and carry a letter/prescription from their health care practitioner that the PAP device is of medical necessity.

Most PAP devices have features to account for variable voltage sources, especially for international travel, and the devices may also have a built-in compensatory mechanism for altitude adjustments. It has been shown that PAP devices at higher altitudes will provide less airflow pressure as a result of the decreased air density.[85] In these circumstances, PAP users may consider wearing an OA as a substitute treatment during travel.

## Sleep apnea in the perioperative period

There is a greater risk of complications from general anesthesia relative to individuals with SRBD. As such, the disorder should be diagnosed and managed prior to the use of general anesthesia. In addition, these same individuals must be closely monitored postoperatively to preclude any SRBD problems. It is not uncommon for individuals with SRBD to bring and use their PAP devices at the hospital during the postoperative period.

# CONCLUSION

PAP is the primary type of therapy for patients with OSA, snoring, and UARS. There are three primary types of PAP modes: CPAP, BiPAP, and APAP. Flexible CPAP is a more recent development as a possible fourth PAP mode.

PAP creates a "pneumatic splint" that maintains upper airway patency, thereby improving the continuity and quality of sleep as well as the overall quality of life for individuals diagnosed with OSA. Studies have demonstrated the effectiveness of PAP for the management of OSA.

The significant challenge to successful PAP therapy, however, is adherence (compliance) since individuals can experience adverse side effects as well as difficulties tolerating the airflow pressure. PAP therapy is usually effective if used on a regular basis.

# REFERENCES

1. Loube DI, Gay PC, Strohl KP, et al. Indications for positive airway pressure treatment of adult obstructive sleep apnea patients: a consensus statement. Chest. 1999; 115(3):863–866.
2. Kushida CA, Littner MR, Hirshkowitz M, et al. American Academy of Sleep Medicine. Practice parameters for the use of continuous and bilevel positive airway pressure devices to treat adult patients with sleep-related breathing disorders. Sleep. 2006; 29(3):375–380.
3. Gay P, Weaver T, Loube D, et al. Evaluation of positive airway pressure treatment for sleep related breathing disorders in adults. Sleep. 2006; 29:381–401.
4. Engelman HM and Wild MR. Improving CPAP use by patients with the sleep apnea/hypopnea syndrome. Sleep Med Rev. 2003; 7:81–99.
5. Pack AI and Maislin G. Who should get treated for sleep apnea? Ann Intern Med. 2001; 134:1065–1066.
6. George CF. Reduction in motor-vehicle collisions following treatment of sleep apnea with nasal CPAP. Thorax. 2001; 56:508–512.
7. He J, Kryger MH, Zorick FJ, et al. Mortality and apnea index in obstructive sleep apnea. Chest. 1988; 94:9–14.

8. Pepperd PE, Young T, Palta M, et al. Prospective study of the association between sleep-disordered breathing and hypertension. N Engl J Med. 2000; 342:1378–1384.

9. Peker Y, Hedner J, Norum J, et al. Increased incidence of cardiovascular disease in middle-aged men with obstructive sleep apnea: a 7-year follow-up. Am J Respir Crit Care Med. 2002; 166:159–165.

10. Nieto FJ, Young TB, Lind BK, et al. Association of sleep-disordered breathing, sleep apnea, and hypertension in a large community based study. Sleep Heart Health Study. J Am Med Assoc. 2000; 283(14):1829–1985.

11. Shahar E, Whitney CW, Redline S, et al. Sleep disordered breathing and cardiovascular disease: cross-sectional results of the Sleep Heart Health Study. Am J Respir Crit Care Med. 2001; 163:19–25.

12. Becker HF, Jerrentrup A, Plock T, et al. Effect of nasal continuous positive airway pressure treatment on blood pressure in obstructive sleep apnea. Circulation. 2003; 107(1):68–73.

13. Beninati W, Harris CD, Herold DL, et al. The effect of snoring and obstructive sleep apnea on sleep quality of bed partners. Mayo Clin Proc. 1999; 74:955–958.

14. Young T, Peppard P, Palta M, et al. Population-based study of sleep-disordered breathing as a risk factor for hypertension. Arch Intern Med. 1997; 157(15):1746–1752.

15. Center for Medicare and Medicaid Services. Medicare Coverage Issues Manual. Transmittal 151, Continuous Positive Airway Pressure (CPAP). January 14, 2002; 60–71.

16. Abbey NC, Cooper KR, and Kwentus JA. Benefit of nasal CPAP in obstructive sleep apnea is due to positive pharyngeal pressure. Sleep. 1989; 12(5):420–422.

17. Series F, Cormier Y, Couture J, et al. Changes in upper airway resistance with lung inflation and positive airway pressure. J Appl Physiol. 1990; 68(3):1075–1079.

18. Kuna ST, Bedi DG, and Ryckman C. Effect of nasal airway positive pressure on upper airway size and configuration. Am Rev Respir Dis. 1988; 138:969–975.

19. Abbey NC, Block AJ, Green D, et al. Measurement of pharyngeal volume by digitized magnetic resonance imaging: effect of nasal continuous positive airway pressure. Am Rev Respir Dis. 1989; 140:717–723.

20. Schwab RJ, Pack AI, Gupta KB, et al. Upper airway and soft tissue structural changes influences by CPAP in normal subjects. Am J Respir Crit Care Med. 1996; 154:1106–1116.

21. Alex CG, Aronson RM, Onal E, et al. Effects of continuous positive airway pressure on upper airway and respiratory muscle activity. J Appl Physiol. 1987; 62:2026–2030.

22. Strohl KP and Redline S. Nasal CPAP therapy, upper airway muscle activation and obstructive sleep apnea. Am Rev Respir Dis. 1986; 134:555–558.

23. Pepin JL, Krieger J, Rodenstein D, et al. Effective compliance during the first three months of continuous positive airway pressure. A European

prospective study of 121 patients. Am J Respir Crit Care Med. 1999; 160(4):1124–1129.

24. Kribbs NB, Pack AI, Kline LR, et al. Objective measurement of patterns of nasal CPAP use by patients with obstructive sleep apnea. Am J Respir Crit Care Med. 1993; 147:887–895.

25. Weaver TE, Kribbs NB, Pack AI, et al. Night to night variability in CPAP use over the first three months of treatment. Sleep. 1997; 20:278–283.

26. Weaver TE, Laizner A, Evans L, et al. An instrument to measure functional status outcomes for disorders of excessive sleepiness. Sleep. 1997; 20(10):835–843.

27. Dinges DF, Pack F, Williams K, et al. Cumulative sleepiness, mood disturbance, and psychomotor vigilance performance decrements during a week of sleep restricted to 4–5 hours per night. Sleep. 1997; 20:276–277.

28. Stepnowsky C and Moore P. Nasal CPAP treatment for obstructive sleep apnea: developing a new perspective on dosing strategies and compliance. J Psychosom Res. 2003; 54:599–605.

29. Massie CA, Hart RW, Peralez K, et al. Effects of humidification on nasal symptoms and compliance in sleep apnea patients using continuous positive airway pressure. Chest. 1999; 116(2):403–408.

30. Rakotonanahary D, Pelletier-Fleury N, Gagnadoux F, et al. Predictive factors for the need for additional humidification during nasal continuous positive airway pressure therapy. Chest. 2001; 119(2):460–465.

31. Sin D, Mayers I, Man G, et al. Long-term compliance rates to continuous positive airway pressure in obstructive sleep apnea: a population-based study. Chest. 2002; 121(2):430–435.

32. Lewis K, Seale L, Bartle I, et al. Early predictors of CPAP use for the treatment of obstructive sleep apnea. Sleep. 2004; 27(1):134–138.

33. Stepnowsky C, Bardwell W, Moore P, et al. Psychologic correlates of compliance with continuous positive airway pressure. Sleep. 2002; 25(7):758–762.

34. Popescu G, Latham M, Allgar V, et al. Continuous positive airway pressure for sleep apnea/hypopnea syndrome: usefulness of a 2 week trial to identify factors associated with long term use. Thorax. 2001; 56(9): 727–733.

35. Richards GN, Cistulli PA, Ungar RG, et al. Mouth leak with nasal continuous positive airway pressure increases nasal airway resistance. Am J Respir Crit Care Med. 1996; 154(1):182–186.

36. Sanders MH and Kern N. Obstructive sleep apnea treated by independently adjusted inspiratory and expiratory positive airway pressures via nasal mask. Chest. 1990; 98:317–324.

37. Littner M, Hirshkowitz M, Davila D, et al. Practice parameters for the use of auto-titrating continuous positive airway pressure devices for titrating pressures and treating adult patients with obstructive sleep apnea syndrome. An American Academy of Sleep Medicine report. Sleep. 2002; 25(2):143–147.

38. Berry RB, Parish JM, and Hartse KM. The use of auto-titrating continuous positive airway pressure for treatment of adult obstructive sleep apnea.

An American Academy of Sleep Medicine review. Sleep. 2002; 25(2):148–173.

39. Teschler H and Berthon-Jones M. Intelligent CPAP systems: clinical experience. Thorax. 1998; 53:S49–S54.

40. Aloia MS, Stanchina M, Arnedt JT, et al. Treatment adherence and outcomes in flexible vs standard continuous positive airway pressure therapy. Chest. 2005; 172:2085–2093.

41. Sullivan CE, Issa FG, Berthon-Jones M, et al. Reversal of obstructive sleep apnea by continuous positive airway pressure applied throughout the nares. Lancet. 1981; 1:862–865.

42. Ficker JH, Wiest GH, Lehnert G, et al. Evaluation of an auto-CPAP device for treatment of obstructive sleep apnea. Thorax. 1998; 53:643–648.

43. Lloberes P, Ballester E, Montserrat JM, et al. Comparison of manual and automatic CPAP titration in patients with sleep apnea/hyponea syndrome. Am J Respir Crit Care Med. 1996; 154:1755–1758.

44. Lofaso F, Lorino AM, Duizabo D, et al. Evaluation of an auto-CPAP device based on snoring detection. Eur Respir J. 1996; 9:1795–1800.

45. Randerath W, Parys K, Feldmeyer F, et al. Self-adjusting continuous positive airway pressure therapy based on the measurement of impedence—a comparison of two different maximum pressure levels. Chest. 1999; 116:991–999.

46. Criner GJ, Brennan K, Travaline JM, et al. Efficacy and compliance with noninvasive positive airway pressure ventilation in patients with chronic respiratory failure. Chest. 1994; 116(3):667–675.

47. Gay PC, Herold DL, and Olson EJ. A randomized, double-blind clinical trial comparing continuous positive airway pressure with a novel bilevel pressure system for treatment of obstructive sleep apnea syndrome. Sleep. 2003; 26(7):864–869.

48. Stauffer JL, Fayter NA, and MacLurg BJ. Conjunctivitis from nasal CPAP apparatus. Chest. 1984; 86:802.

49. Berry RB and Block AJ. Positive nasal airway pressure eliminated snoring as well as obstructive sleep apnea. Chest. 1984; 85:15–20.

50. Sanders MH. Nasal CPAP effect on patterns of sleep apnea. Chest. 1984; 86:839–844.

51. Rappaport DM, Sorkin B, Garay SM, et al. Reversal of the "Pickwickian Syndrome" by long-term use of nocturnal nasal airway pressure. N Engl J Med. 1982; 931–933.

52. Prosise GL and Berry RB. Oral-nasal continuous positive airway pressure as a treatment for obstructive sleep apnea. Chest. 1994; 106:180–186.

53. Sanders MH, Kern NB, Stiller RA, et al. CPAP therapy via oronasal mask for obstructive sleep apnea. Chest. 1994; 106:774–779.

54. Mortimore IL, Whittle AT, and Douglas NJ. Comparison of nose and face mask CPAP therapy for sleep apnea. Thorax. 1998; 53:290–292.

55. Powell NB, Zonato AI, Weaver AM, et al. Radiofrequency treatment of turbinate hypertrophy in subjects using continuous positive airway pressure: a randomized, double-blind, placebo-controlled clinical pilot trial. Laryngoscope. 2001; 111:1783–1790.

56. Young T, Palta M, Dempsey J, et al. The occurrence of sleep-disordered breathing among middle-aged adults. N Engl J Med. 1993; 328(17):1230–1235.

57. Cheson A. American Sleep Disorders Standard of Practice Committee, Chairman. Practice parameters for the indications for polysomnography and related procedures. Sleep. 1997; 20(6):406–422.

58. Pevernagie DA and Sheard JW Jr. Relations between sleep stage, posture and effective nasal CPAP levels in OSA. Sleep. 1992; 15:162–167.

59. Neill AM, Angus SM, Sajkov D, et al. Effects of sleep posture on upper airway stability in patients with obstructive sleep apnea. Am J Respir Crit Care Med. 1997; 155:199–204.

60. Oksenberg A, Silverberg DS, Arons E, et al. The sleep supine position has a major effect on optimal nasal continuous positive airway pressure: relationship with rapid eye movements and non-rapid eye movements sleep, body mass index, respiratory disturbance index, and age. Chest. 1999; 116(4):1000–1006.

61. Schwartz AR, Gold AR, Schubert N, et al. Effect of weight loss on upper airway collapsibility in obstructive sleep apnea. Am Rev Respir Dis. 1991; 144:494–498.

62. Jenkinson C, Davies RJO, Mullins R, et al. Comparison of therapeutic and subtherapeutic nasal continuous positive airway pressure for obstructive sleep apnea: a randomized prospective parallel trial. Lancet. 1999; 353:2100–2105.

63. Ballester E, Badia JR, Hernandex L, et al. Evidence of the effectiveness of continuous positive airway pressure in the treatment of sleep apnea/hypopnea syndrome. Am J Respir Crit Care Med. 1999; 159:495–501.

64. Sin DD, Mayers I, Man GC, et al. Can continuous positive airway pressure therapy improve the general health status of patients with obstructive sleep apnea? A clinical effectiveness study. Chest. 2002; 122:1679–1685.

65. Weaver T, Maislin G, Dinges D, et al. Relationship between hours of CPAP use and achieving normal levels of sleepiness and daily functioning. Sleep. 2007; 30:711–719.

66. Marshall N, Barnes M, Travier N, et al. Continuous positive airway pressure reduces daytime sleepiness in mild to moderate obstructive sleep apnea: a meta-analysis. Thorax. 2006; 61:430–434.

67. Patel S, White D, Malhotra A, et al. Continuous positive airway pressure therapy for treating sleepiness in a diverse population with obstructive sleep apnea: results of a meta-analysis. Arch Intern Med. 2003; 163:565–571.

68. Rajagopal KR, Bennet LL, Dillard TA, et al. Overnight nasal CPAP improves hypersomnolence in sleep apnea. Chest. 1986; 90:172–176.

69. Campos-Rodriguez E, Perez-Ronchel J, Grilo-Reina A, et al. Long-term effect of continuous positive airway pressure on BP in patients with hypertension and sleep apnea. Chest. 2007; 132:1847–1852.

70. Akashiba T, Minemura H, Yamamoto H, et al. Nasal continuous positive airway pressure changes blood pressure "non-dippers" to "dippers" in patients with obstructive sleep apnea. Sleep. 1999; 22:849–853.

71. Hla KM, Skatrud JB, Finn L, et al. The effect of sleep-disordered breathing on BP in untreated hypertension. Chest. 2002; 122(4):1125–1132.

72. Faccenda J, Mackay TM, Boon NA, et al. Randomized placebo-controlled trial of continuous positive airway pressure on blood pressure in the sleep apnea-hypopnea syndrome. Am J Respir Crit Care Med. 2001; 163(2):344–348.

73. Engleman HE, Kingshott RH, Wraith PK, et al. Randomized placebo-controlled crossover trial of continuous positive airways pressure for mild obstructive apnea/hypopnea syndrome. Am J Respir Crit Care Med. 1999; 159(2):461–467.

74. Redline S, Adams N, Strauss ME, et al. Improvement of mild sleep-disordered breathing with CPAP compared with conservative therapy. Am J Respir Crit Care Med. 1998; 157(3 Pt 1):858–865.

75. Montserrat JM, Ferrer M, Hernandez L, et al. Effectiveness of CPAP treatment in daytime function in sleep apnea syndrome: a randomized controlled study with an optimized placebo. Am J Respir Crit Care Med. 2001; 164(4):608–613.

76. Schwartz D, Kohler W, and Karatinos G. Symptoms of depression in individuals with obstructive sleep apnea may be amenable to treatment with continuous positive airway pressure. Chest. 2005; 128:1304–1309.

77. Findley I, Smith C, Hooper J, et al. Treatment with nasal CPAP decreases automobile accidents in patients with sleep apnea. Am J Respir Crit Care Med. 2000; 161:857–859.

78. Engleman HM, Marin SE, and Douglas NJ. Compliance with CPAP therapy in patients with the sleep apnea-hypopnea syndrome. Thorax. 1994; 49:263–266.

79. Pepin JL, Leger P, Veale D, et al. Side effects of nasal continuous positive airway pressure in sleep apnea syndrome. Study of 193 patients in two French sleep centers. Chest. 1995; 107(2):375–381.

80. Rolfe I, Olson LG, and Sanders NA. Long-term acceptance of continuous positive airway pressure in obstructive sleep apnea. Am Rev Respir Dis. 1991; 144:1130–1133.

81. Meurice JC, Marc I, Carrier G, et al. Effects of mouth opening on upper airway collapsibility in normal sleeping subjects. Am J Respir Crit Care Med. 1996; 153:255–259.

82. Friedman M, Tanyeri H, Lim JW, et al. Effect of improved nasal breathing on obstructive sleep apnea. Otolaryng Head Neck Surg. 2000; 122:71–74.

83. Martins de Araujo MT, Vieira SD, Vasquez EC, et al. Heated humidification or face mask to prevent upper airway dryness during continuous positive airway pressure therapy. Chest. 2000; 117:142–147.

84. Sanner BM, Fluerenbrock N, Kleiber-Imback A, et al. Effect of continuous positive airway pressure therapy on infectious complications in patients with obstructive sleep apnea syndrome. Respiration. 2001; 68:483–487.

85. Fromm RE Jr, Varon J, Lechin AE, et al. CPAP machine performance and altitude. Chest. 1995; 108:1577–1580.

# 10

# Surgical treatment for sleep-related breathing disorders

## CONCEPTUAL OVERVIEW

The *International Classification of Sleep Disorders-2* (*ICSD-2*) regards sleep-related breathing disorders (SRBD) as being "characterized by disordered respiration during sleep."[1] A subcategory of SRBD is obstructive sleep apnea (OSA). In order to effectively treat OSA, it is imperative to assess which of the upper airway structures are contributory to the diagnosed disorder.

The upper airway can be regarded as being composed of three anatomical zones[2] (Figures 10.1 and 10.2):

1. The nasopharynx (i.e., the nasal turbinates to the hard palate)
2. The oropharynx that includes both the retropalatal area (i.e., the hard palate to the caudal marging of the soft palate) and the retroglossal area (i.e., the caudal margin of the soft palate to the epiglottis)
3. The hypopharynx (i.e., the base of the tongue to the larynx)

Although obstruction of the upper airway may include multiple anatomical sites, closure of the upper airway is most commonly located in the retropalatal and retroglossal areas (Figures 10.3–10.5).[2] Vibration of the airflow past the pharyngeal soft tissues can result in snoring, and a narrowing or collapse of the upper airway may result in obstructive respiratory disturbances during sleep, such as hypopnea or apnea. Surgery of the upper airway may be considered as a management option, especially for patients for whom treatment involving positive airway pressure (PAP) therapy or oral appliance (OA) therapy is not effective or tolerable.

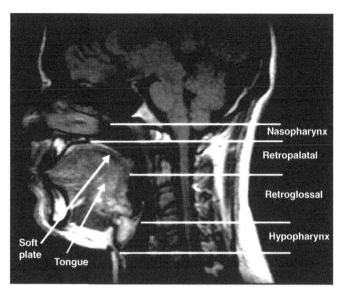

**Figure 10.1** Midsagittal MRI of a normal subject. It indicates the regions of the upper airway. (Schwab R. Imaging for the snoring and sleep apnea patient. In: Attanasio R and Bailey D, eds. Sleep Disorders: Dentistry's Role (Dental Clinics of North America, 45:4). Philadelphia: W.B. Saunders. 2001; 761. Reprinted with permission.)

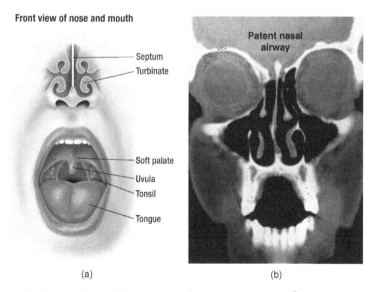

(a)  (b)

**Figure 10.2** (a) Normal frontal view of the upper airway. (© Krames Medical Publishing, 2009. Used with permission.) (b) Coronal CT scan of a normal airway with clear paranasal sinuses, relatively straight septum, and normal turbinates, resulting in a patent nasal airway. (Aragon S. Surgical management for snoring and sleep apnea. In: Attanasio R and Bailey D, eds. Sleep Disorders: Dentistry's Role (Dental Clinics of North America, 45:4). Philadelphia: W.B. Saunders. 2001; 868. Reprinted with permission.)

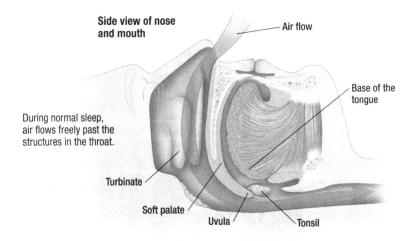

**Figure 10.3**    Normal sagittal view of the upper airway. (© Krames Medical Publishing, 2009. Used with permission).

The goal of this chapter is to provide an overview of the more common types of surgical intervention techniques that are employed for the management of snoring and OSA.

# INDICATIONS FOR SURGICAL INTERVENTION

The purpose of surgical intervention is to improve airway patency during sleep by enlarging the upper airway and correction of any disproportionate anatomy.

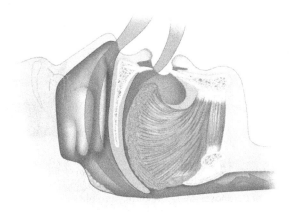

**Figure 10.4**    Sagittal view of partially blocked upper airway. (© Krames Medical Publishing, 2009. Used with permission.)

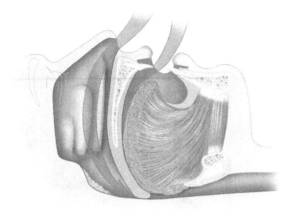

**Figure 10.5**    Sagittal view of completely blocked upper airway. (© Krames Medical Publishing, 2009. Used with permission.)

Surgery is indicated (1) after unsuccessful nonsurgical conservative therapeutic interventions such as PAP, behavioral approaches (e.g., weight loss, sleep hygiene), and OA; or (2) when an abnormal soft tissue structure is identified as being responsible for the OSA.[3]

It has been shown that only a very small percentage of patients with OSA have a readily identifiable anatomical area of narrowing or collapse that contributes to the upper airway resistance or collapse.[4] Most OSA patients present with a diffuse soft tissue blockage or disproportionate anatomical component of the upper airway that is not always readily observable,[4] and thus warrants a complete evaluation.

## PRESURGICAL EVALUATION

The purpose of the presurgical evaluation is to identify site-specific areas in the upper airway that contribute to or cause the OSA. These findings become part of the process of determining which surgical approach, if any, is warranted to address the anatomical obstruction.

Because different areas of the upper airway may be involved in the etiology of the SRBD, a complete patient evaluation is necessary to (1) assess the probable areas of anatomical involvement in airway narrowing or collapse and (2) determine if any existing pathologies such as neoplasms or cysts are present. Most common clinical findings associated with OSA are disproportionate anatomy such as a large or elongated soft palate (Figure 10.6), a thickened or elongated uvula (Figure 10.7), an enlarged tongue particularly at the base (Figure 10.8), a deviated nasal septum (Figures 10.9 and 10.10), nasal turbinates that are hypertrophic (Figures 10.10 and 10.11),

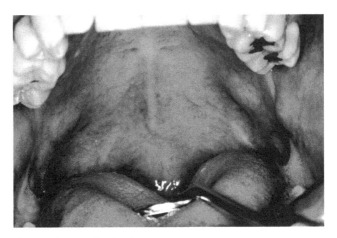

**Figure 10.6**    Elongated palatal tissue.

presence of nasal polyps (Figure 10.12), and a hypoplastic or retrognathic mandible.

Ideally included in the evaluation is a polysomnogram (PSG) to help determine the extent of the breathing disorder, a comprehensive history, and a comprehensive head and neck clinical examination that includes a nasopharyngolaryngeal examination through the use of a flexible fiberoptic endoscope. The findings from the clinical examination can also be complemented by imaging studies (e.g., cephalometrics, magnetic resonance imaging (MRI), computed tomography (CT) scan).[5]

The outcomes of an ideal presurgical clinical examination would serve as predictors for the locations of any narrowed or collapsed areas of the upper airway. Unfortunately, because of its subjective nature, clinical

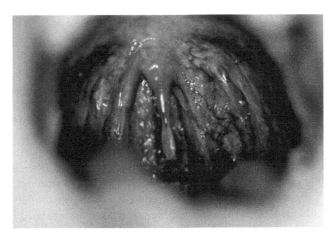

**Figure 10.7**    Elongated uvula.

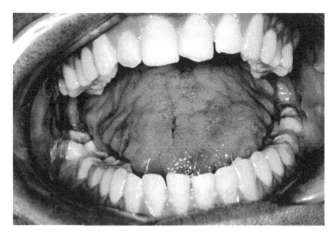

**Figure 10.8**    Enlarged tongue.

examination in and of itself is insufficient for complete assessment of the upper airway in identification of SRBD.[6] In addition, clinical examinations, including the use of fiberoptic endoscopy, are generally conducted when the patient is not in a true sleep state.

Although the literature does not provide a definitive means of establishing a predictive value regarding which patients would benefit from all surgical techniques,[7–9] there have been two classification systems typically used during clinical examinations with respect to pharyngeal anatomy. The

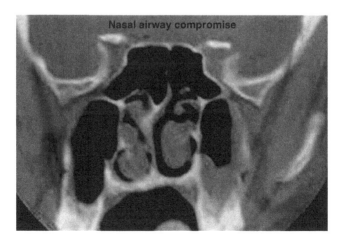

**Figure 10.9**    Coronal CT scan of an impaired nasal airway because of pansinusitis leading to purulent rhinosinusitis. (Aragon S. Surgical management for snoring and sleep apnea. In: Attanasio R and Bailey D, eds. Sleep Disorders: Dentistry's Role (Dental Clinics of North America, 45:4). Philadelphia: W.B. Saunders. 2001; 869. Reprinted with permission.)

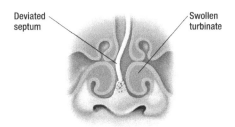

Air may not be able to move freely past
a deviated septum or swollen turbinates.

**Figure 10.10**   Frontal view of the upper airway demonstrating a deviated septum and swollen turbinates. (© Krames Medical Publishing, 2009. Used with permission.)

first, known as the Mallampati classification, was based on palate position, and it was used as a prognostic indicator relative to the potential difficulties of tracheal intubation.[10] Two other clinical staging systems for SRBD were subsequently developed, known as the Friedman classifications, related to tongue position and tonsil size with respect to the palate[11,12] (Figures 10.13 and 10.14). The Friedman tongue position classification has been investigated as a prognostic indicator for the presence and severity of obstruction in the hypopharynx region.[13]

Incorporating a classification with respect to position of the tongue, tonsils, and palate into a complete head and neck examination is warranted

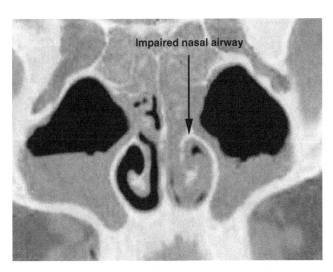

**Figure 10.11**   Coronal CT scan of a compromised nasal airway because of marked septal deviation, turbinate hypertrophy, and maxillary sinusitis. (Aragon S. Surgical management for snoring and sleep apnea. In: Attanasio R and Bailey D, eds. Sleep Disorders: Dentistry's Role (Dental Clinics of North America, 45:4). Philadelphia: W.B. Saunders. 2001; 869. Reprinted with permission.)

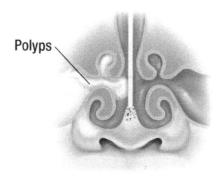

**Figure 10.12**    Frontal view of the upper airway demonstrating polyps. (© Krames Medical Publishing, 2009. Used with permission.)

for any patient prior to undergoing any surgical intervention for snoring and OSA since the findings may direct the surgeon in the selection and site of surgical treatment.

# TYPES OF SURGERY

On the basis of the outcomes of the presurgical evaluation, surgical treatment is site-specific. There are a variety of surgical procedures available, ranging from minimally invasive to more invasive. The purpose of the minimally invasive procedures is to obtain relatively small changes in the structures and biomechanics of the upper airway, whereas the more invasive procedures are meant to achieve significant removal of tissues and sometimes also a repositioning of anatomical structures (e.g., advancement of the mandible and/or maxilla).

## Tracheostomy

Tracheostomy was the first surgical procedure introduced for the treatment of OSA.[14] However, since the employment of PAP therapy and other surgical procedures, tracheostomy is no longer the standard surgical treatment for OSA.[15] Also, when compared with PAP therapy and the other surgical procedures, tracheostomy is regarded to have adverse psychological, social, and esthetic effects.

This procedure completely bypasses any obstruction in the upper airway because it is performed distal to both the larynx and the pharynx. As such, this procedure has been demonstrated to result in significant improvement of OSA.[16]

Despite the aforementioned adverse effects, tracheostomy is still indicated when (1) the severe OSA is life-threatening from an immediate

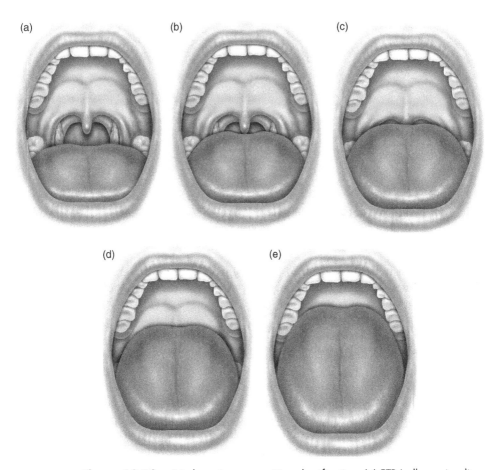

**Figure 10.13**    Friedman tongue position classification. (a) FTP I allows visualization of the entire uvula and tonsils/pillars. (b) FTP IIa allows visualization of most of the uvula, but the tonsils/pillars are absent. (c) FTP IIb allows visualization of the entire soft palate to the base of the uvula. (d) FTP III allows visualization of some of the soft palate, but the distal structures are absent. (e) FTP IV allows visualization of the hard palate only. (Friedman M, Soans R, Gurpinar B, et al. Interexaminer agreement of Friedman tongue positions for staging of obstructive sleep apnea/hypopnea syndrome. Otolaryngol Head Neck Surg. 2008; 139:373. Reprinted with permission.)

obstruction or associated with significant comorbidity, (2) PAP therapy is either not tolerated or it does not address the severe deoxygenation, and (3) airway control is needed during upper airway reconstruction.

## Nasal surgery

Even though narrowing and collapse of the upper airway occur mostly in the retropalatal and retroglossal areas, the nasal portion of the upper

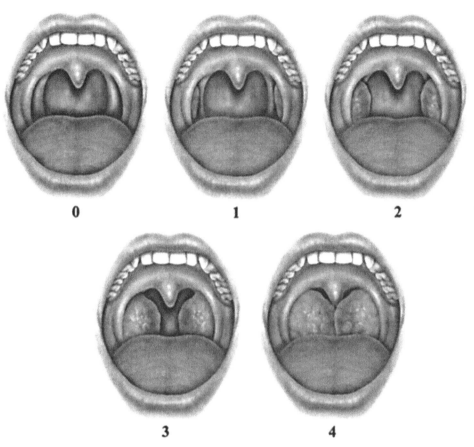

**Figure 10.14** Tonsil size is graded from 0 to 4. Tonsil size 0 denotes surgically removed tonsils. Size 1 implies tonsils hidden within the pillars. Tonsil size 2 implies the tonsils extending to the pillars. Size 3 tonsils are beyond the pillars but not to the midline. Tonsil size 4 implies tonsils extended to the midline. (Friedman M, Ibrahim H, Lee G, et al. Combined uvulopalatalpharyngoplasty and radiofrequency tongue base reduction for treatment of obstructive sleep apnea/hypopnea syndrome. Otolaryngol Head Neck Surg. 2003; 129(6):614. Reprinted with permission.)

airway can have a significant effect on these sites. One of the functions of the nasal airway is to allow for a level of resistance in the upper airway. If there is an increase in the level of resistance in the nasal airway, there can be a related increase in pharyngeal negative pressure that may contribute to the narrowing and even obstruction of the airway in the velopharyngeal and hypopharyngeal areas.[5]

Impaired nasal breathing can result in individuals who are sensitized from exposure to high allergens or in individuals suffering from rhinitis. This experience of impaired nasal breathing during sleep can result in poor sleep quality and excessive daytime sleepiness. It is not uncommon during sleep for nasal congestion to cause an individual to mouth breathe, and therefore rotating the mandible down and back. When this occurs, the base of the tongue can narrow the airway space in the pharynx. Thus, nasal airflow resistance could have an impact on the severity of SRBD.[17,18]

Investigations have demonstrated that sleep quality worsened with experimental nasal occlusion.[19-21] Individuals are at greater risk for developing SRBD if they have rhinitis and nasal congestion during sleep,[22,23] severe septal deviation or inferior turbinate hypertrophy,[24,25] and nasal polyposis.[26]

The primary purpose of nasal surgery is to improve the patency of the nasal airway which can subsequently improve SRBD.[24,27-29] However, the rate of success for nasal surgery is regarded as low when success is defined as a $\geq$50% reduction of AHI (apnea–hypopnea index) and <20 AHI score. One study demonstrated a worsening of the OSA by a surgical correction procedure of a deviated septum.[30] At times, the purpose of the nasal surgery may only be to improve the compliance of using PAP by providing the patient with a clear nasal airway. Thus, the indications for nasal surgery include obstruction of airflow from deviation of the septum, enlarged turbinates, nasal polyps, or narrowing of the nasal valve.

The more common nasal surgeries include septoplasty, turbinoplasty, turbinectomy, polypectomy, adenoidectomy, and enlargement of the nasal valve.

## Tonsillectomy

It is not uncommon for hypertrophic palatine tonsillar tissues to be responsible for obstruction in the posterior pharyngeal region of the airway. Using the definition of surgical success as >50% reduction of AHI and <20 AHI score, tonsillectomy has been demonstrated to be effective in 80% of adults with severe OSA and 100% effective in adults with mild OSA.[31] Although tonsillectomy and adenoidectomy are primarily performed in children, tonsillectomy is regarded as an accepted treatment modality for adults with OSA.[32]

In an effort to lessen the degree of postoperative discomfort that can accompany the surgical or electrical cautery excision of tonsillar tissue, tissue ablation through the use of temperature-controlled radio frequency has been shown to be effective.[33,34]

## Uvulopalatopharyngoplasty

The most common surgical procedure for increasing the oropharyngeal airway space is the uvulopalatopharyngoplasty (UPPP). This procedure was initially described in 1964 as a surgical means of addressing snoring, and it was later modified to also address OSA.[1,35,36] UPPP involves reduction of tissues in the areas of the soft palate, uvula, and the lateral and posterior

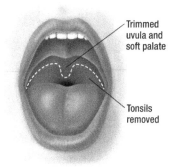

Trimmed
uvula and
soft palate

Tonsils
removed

UPPP trims the uvula and removes
other tissue from the back of the mouth.

**Figure 10.15**    Depiction of UPPP surgical procedure. (© Krames Medical Publishing, 2009. Used with permission.)

walls of the pharynx (Figures 10.15–10.17).[37] It is common for a tonsillectomy to be performed at the same time as the UPPP.

The degree of removal of soft tissues can vary and is dependent on the site-specific issues of each patient. The more radical UPPP procedure does not necessarily equate to more effectiveness, but it can lead to increased complications. The more common postoperative complications can include surgery-associated pain, infection, velopharyngeal insufficiency, speech disturbance, and nasopharyngeal stenosis. Nonetheless, UPPP is regarded as a safe surgical procedure.[38]

As with the other surgical procedures, the criteria for success include a ≥50% reduction of the AHI and a <20 AHI score. The success rate for treatment of OSA can range from 25 to 75%.[39–44] The more the obstruction

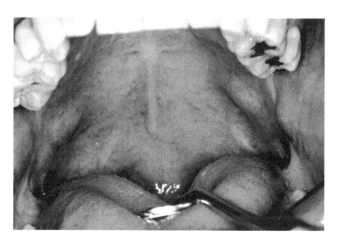

**Figure 10.16**    Pre-UPPP: elongated palatal tissue.

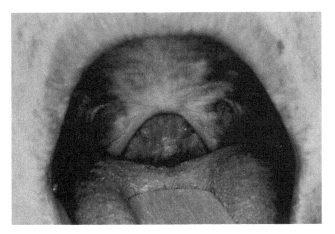

**Figure 10.17**    Post-UPPP.

is limited to the retropalatal area, the greater the success rate. The most common reason for reduction in the success rate is the presence of anatomical obstruction in the retroglossal or hypopharyngeal area, for example the base of the tongue[45] or other tissues.[46] One study demonstrated that the Friedman classifications for palate position and tonsil size were a valuable prognostic indicator for UPPP successful outcomes.[12]

## Tongue-base suspension

Even though OSA patients often have multiple sites of obstruction or narrowing of the airway,[36] the most common anatomical areas with obstruction are the base of the tongue and the retroglossal areas.[47] When the base of the tongue may be identified as the primary site of obstruction, a tongue-base suspension (TBS) surgical procedure can be indicated (Figure 10.18).

To help counterbalance the collapse of the base of the tongue in the hypopharynx, a permanent suture is looped through the base of the tongue and attached to a titanium screw that has been placed in the geniotubercle portion of the mandible. The tension of the suture decreases the collapsibility of the base of the tongue against the posterior wall of the pharynx during sleep.[47,48] This procedure may result in a "tongue base dimple due to the suspension suture"[49] (Figure 10.19).

There is a low success rate of 20% with this procedure.[50] However, when TBS is combined with UPPP, the success rate significantly increases to above 80% in patients with severe OSA.[49]

## Surgical reduction of the tongue

A more radical surgical procedure for an enlarged base of the tongue occluding the retroglossal area is the surgical reduction of the posterior aspect

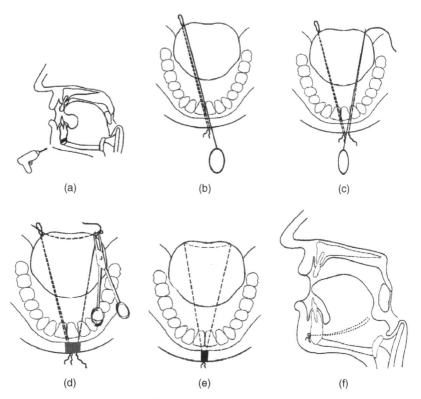

(a)                         (b)                         (c)

(d)                         (e)                         (f)

**Figure 10.18**   Schematic illustrations of the operative procedure. (a) Submental incision and the creation of the small hole on the mandible. (b) Passing the silk suture loop to the tongue base with a suture passer. (c) Passing the suture. (d) Passing the suture across the tongue. (e) and (f) Tying the suture on the mandibular hole. (Omur M, Ozturan D, Elez F, et al. Tongue base suspension combined with UPPP in severe OSA patients. Otolaryngol Head Neck Surg. 2005; 133:220. Reprinted with permission.)

of the tongue. This can be accomplished with a midline glossectomy that excises a rectangular portion of the tongue.[51] Another technique is the linguloplasty that is more aggressive in the amount of tissue removal with the postsurgical defect, resulting in an anterior advancement of the base of the tongue. This latter procedure can significantly improve the success rate to 75%.[52]

Because of the significant edema at the surgical site, both surgical procedures necessitate the use of a tracheotomy. Postoperative complications can include difficulty swallowing, disturbed taste, and bleeding.

## Tissue ablation with radio frequency

Radio frequency (RF) for the ablation or removal of soft tissue has been used for the management of a hypertrophic prostrate and other body

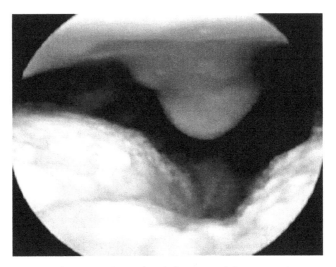

**Figure 10.19**    The tongue base dimple because of the suspension suture. (Omur M, Ozturan D, Elez F, et al. Tongue base suspension combined with UPPP in severe OSA patients. Otolaryngol Head Neck Surg. 2005; 133:220. Reprinted with permission.)

areas. An RF generator produces a low heat energy that can be used to denature tissue protein in the area surrounding the electrode probe without any destruction of surface tissue. RF has been demonstrated in animal studies to be effective in the reduction or ablation of excess or redundant tongue tissue.[53]

As with the other surgical procedures, the success of RF is dependent on the site-specific diagnosis of the tissue obstruction or narrowing in the airway. Palatoplasty with RF therapy reduced snoring in 60–100% of the patients.[54–57] Interestingly, it has been demonstrated that there may be an 11–41% potential for relapse of snoring 12–18 months following initial RF ablation.[53,58] When there is an unsuccessful response to RF of the retropalatal area, potential airway obstructions in the nasal and/or hypopharyngeal areas should be considered.

RF ablation can also be applied to the base of the tongue. In one study of OSA patients for whom UPPP was not successful, the AHI was significantly reduced following RF ablation of the tongue base.[59] Another study of OSA patients who had multisite obstructions of the airway demonstrated that ablation of soft palatal tissue and the base of the tongue with RF significantly reduced the AHI.[60]

Complications of RF ablation can include ulceration, infection, dysfunction of the soft palatal tissues, and velopharyngeal insufficiency.

A more recent technique employs a submucosal minimally invasive lingual excision (SMILE) in which the RF wand is placed within the tongue base to remove tissue inside as compared to the outer surface of the tongue

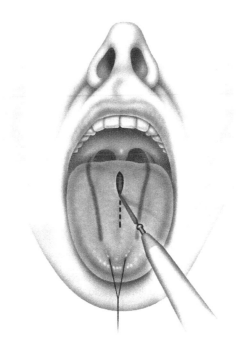

**Figure 10.20**    Midline incision for the SMILE technique. Note the marked course of the lingual arteries on either side of the incision. (Friedman M, Soans R, Gurpinar B, et al. Evaluation of submucosal minimally invasive lingual excision technique for treatment of obstructive sleep apnea/hypopnea syndrome. Otolaryngol Head Neck Surg. 2008; 139:379. Reprinted with permission.)

with the traditional RF approach (Figures 10.20 and 10.21). The results of studies demonstrate significantly increased success rates.[61,62]

## Mandibular osteotomy with genioglossus advancement

Attached to the geniotubercle area of the mandible is the genioglossus muscle of the tongue. A mandibular osteotomy with genioglossus advancement (MOGA) is a surgical procedure that involves the sectioning of a rectangular block of bone surrounding the geniotubercle and advancing that section anterior to the labial surface of the mandible (Figures 10.22–10.25). The outcome is a tension applied to the tongue, which prevents a collapse of the posterior aspect of the tongue into the retroglossal airway during sleep. This technique does not involve any movement of teeth or maxillomandibular osseous structures other than the conservative portion of the geniotubercle.

Expansion of the airway resulting from this procedure has been shown to have a 42–75% success rate.[50,63,64]

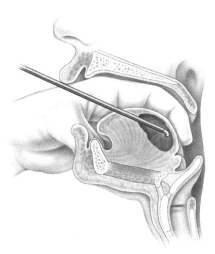

**Figure 10.21**    SMILE technique: coblation wand is introduced through the incision and advanced toward the vallecula. Submucosal tissue excision is guided by palpation with the nondominant hand. (Friedman M, Soans R, Gurpinar B, et al. Evaluation of submucosal minimally invasive lingual excision technique for treatment of obstructive sleep apnea/hypopnea syndrome. Otolaryngol Head Neck Surg. 2008; 139:380. Reprinted with permission.)

## Hyoid myotomy and suspension

Another surgical procedure that results in an expansion of the retroglossal and hypopharyngeal areas is the hyoid myotomy and suspension (HMS). This is particularly effective when there is hypopharyngeal constriction

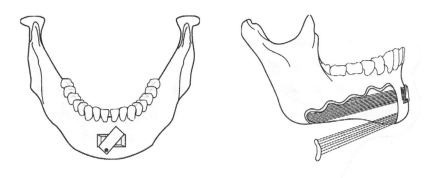

**Figure 10.22**    The genioglossus advancement procedure. A rectangular window of symphyseal bone consisting of the geniotubercle is advanced anteriorly, rotated to allow bony overlap, and immobilized with a titanium screw. (Li KK. Hypopharyngeal airway surgery. Otolaryngol Clin North Am. 2007; 40:848. Reprinted with permission.)

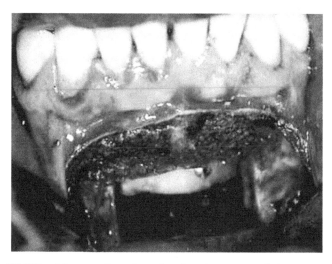

**Figure 10.23**   Intraoperative view showing the extent of the rectangular osteotomy. (Li KK, Riley RW, Powell NB, et al. Obstructive sleep apnea surgery: genioglossus advancement revisited. J Oral Maxillofac Surg. 2001; 59:1183. Reprinted with permission.)

from lateral pharyngeal tissue that is excessive or from an epiglottis that is retrodisplaced.

The procedure involves suspending the hyoid bone over the ala portion of the thyroid via nonresorbable sutures, which should preclude a hypopharyngeal collapse or narrowing since there will be increased tension on the muscles of the tongue (Figure 10.26).

The success rate for this procedure has been shown to vary from 17 to 65%.[46,65–67]

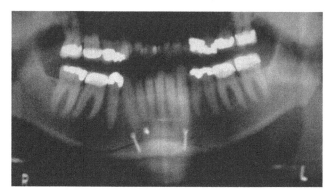

**Figure 10.24**   Panoramic radiograph showing the reconstituted border fixed with two screws. Note the genial tubercle/genioglossus muscle complex (GGC) bone flap is stabilized with a single screw. (Li KK, Riley RW, Powell NB, et al. Obstructive sleep apnea surgery: genioglossus advancement revisited. J Oral Maxillofac Surg. 2001; 59:1184. Reprinted with permission.)

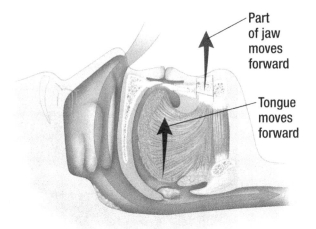

**Figure 10.25**    Depiction of genioglossus advancement surgical procedure. (© Krames Medical Publishing, 2009. Used with permission.)

## Maxillomandibular advancement

A more aggressive surgical procedure involving repositioning of the osseous maxillomandibular components is maxillomandibular advancement (MMA). Although tracheostomy is considered to be the most effective treatment for OSA, MMA is regarded as the next most effective because the procedure involves the retropalatal and retroglossal areas as well as increasing the tension of the genioglossal muscle, thereby significantly improving the airway space[68] (Figure 10.27). Success rate for MMA is 75–100%.[46,58,69,70]

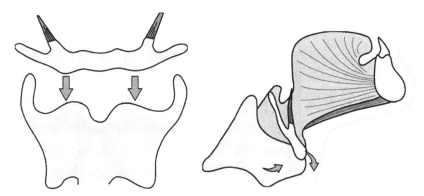

**Figure 10.26**    The hyoid advancement procedure. The hyoid bone is isolated, the inferior body dissected clean, the majority of the suprahyoid musculature remains intact. The hyoid is advanced over the thyroid lamina and immobilized with sutures placed through the superior aspect of the thyroid cartilage. (Li KK. Hypopharyngeal airway surgery. Otolaryngol Clin North Am. 2007; 40:848. Reprinted with permission.)

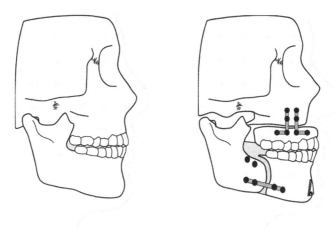

**Figure 10.27**   The maxillomandibular advancement osteotomy procedure. Lefort I maxillary oseotomy with rigid plate fixation and a bilateral sagittal split mandibular osteotomy with bicortical screw fixation. The advancement is at least 10 mm. (Li KK. Hypopharyngeal airway surgery. Otolaryngol Clin North Am. 2007; 40:849. Reprinted with permission.)

Complications of MMA can include long-standing anesthesia or paresthesia, malrelationship of the maxilla and mandible, infection, and bleeding.

## Other considerations

The commercial market has made available two types of expendable devices known as nasal dilators. One is an internal device placed within the nasal passages, and the other is an external nasal strip placed on the outside of the nasal passages. The concept of these devices is to increase the nasal breathing ability by dilation of the nasal valve and thereby decreasing the nasal resistance.[71]

Both have been studied in patients with PSGs.[72–75]

Results demonstrated that although there may be a subjective improvement relative to snoring, the snoring and AHI are not improved for most patients with SRBD.

## CONCLUSION

The gold standard for treating OSA is PAP. However, not all OSA patients are compliant or adhere to the use of a PAP device, and for those individuals there are nonsurgical options, such as OA therapy, or surgical intervention. When considering treatment options, the decisions should be site-specific relative to obstruction or narrowing of the airway spaces.

To determine the site-specific areas of disproportionate anatomy as well as to rule out any pathology of the upper airway, a complete history, clinical evaluation, and appropriate imaging of the patient are necessary.

Surgery is not without its complications, but the patient must weigh the benefits and risks in making the decision when electing to pursue surgery.

# REFERENCES

1. Schwab R. Imaging for the snoring and sleep apnea patient. In: Attanasio R and Bailey D, eds. Sleep Disorders: Dentistry's Role. Philadelphia: W.B. Saunders Co. 2001; 760.
2. Goldberg AN and Schwab RJ. Identifying the patient with sleep apnea: upper airway assessment and physical examination. Otolaryngol Clin North Am. 1998; 31:919–930.
3. Standards of Practice Committee of the American Sleep Disorders Association: Report of the American Sleep Disorders Association. Practice parameters for the treatment of obstructive sleep apnea in adults: the efficacy of surgical modifications of the upper airway. Sleep. 1996; 19(2):152–155.
4. Sher A. Obstructive sleep apnea syndrome: a complex disorder of the upper airway. Otolaryngol Clin North Am. 1990; 23:593–608.
5. Aragon S. Surgical management for snoring and sleep apnea. Dent Clin North Am. 2001; 45(4):867–879.
6. Redline S and Strohl K. Recognition and consequences of obstructive sleep apnea hypopnea syndrome. Otolaryngol Clin North Am. 1999; 32(2): 303–331.
7. Deegan P and McNicholas W. Predictive value of clinical features for the obstructive sleep apnea syndrome. Eur Respir J. 1996; 9(1):117–124.
8. Pradhan P, Glikllich R, and Winkelman J. Screening for obstructive sleep apnea in patients presenting for snoring surgery. Laryngoscope. 1996; 106(11):1393–1397.
9. Tsai W, Remmers J, Brant R, et al. A decision rule for diagnostic testing in obstructive sleep apnea. Am J Respir Crit Care Med. 2003; 167(10):1427–1432.
10. Mallampati SR, Gatt SP, Gugino LD, et al. A clinical sign to predict difficult traceal intubation: a prospective study. Can J Anaesth. 1985; 32:429–434.
11. Friedman M, Tanyeri H, LaRosa M, et al. Clinical predictors of obstructive sleep apnea. Laryngoscope. 1999; 109:1901–1907.
12. Friedman M, Ibrahim H, and Bass L. Clinical staging for sleep-disordered breathing. Otolaryngol Head Neck Surg. 2002; 127:13–21.
13. Friedman M, Soans R, Gurpinar B, et al. Interexaminer agreement of Friedman tongue positions for staging of obstructive sleep apnea/hypopnea syndrome. Otolaryngol Head Neck Surg. 2008; 139:372–377.

14. Kuhl W, Doll E, and Frank M. Erfolgreiche Behandlung eines Pickwick Syndroms durch eine Dauer-trachealkanule. Dtsh Med Wochenschr. 1969; 94:1286–1290.

15. Riley R, Powell N, Guilleminault C, et al. Maxillary, mandibular and hyoid advancement: an alternative to tracheostomy in obstructive sleep apnea syndrome. Otolaryngol Head Neck Surg. 1986; 94:584–588.

16. Campanini A, De Vito A, Frassineti A, et al. Role of skin-lined tracheotomy in obstructive sleep apnea syndrome: personal experience. Acta Otorhinolaryngol Ital. 2004; 24(2):68–74.

17. Rappai M, Collop N, Kemp S, and deShazo R. The nose and sleep-disordered breathing. What we know and what we do not know. Chest. 2003; 124:2309–2323.

18. Cole P and Haight JS. Mechanisms of nasal obstruction in sleep. Laryngoscope. 1984; 94:1557–1559.

19. Lavie P, Fishel N, Zomer J, and Eliashar I. The effects of partial and complete mechanical occlusion of the nasal passages on sleep architecture and breathing in sleep. Acta Otolaryngol. 1985; 95:161–166.

20. Olsen KD, Kern EB, and Westbrook PR. Sleep and breathing disturbances secondary to nasal obstruction. Otolaryngol Head Neck Surg. 1981; 89:804–810.

21. Surrat PM, Turner BL, and Wilhoit SC. Effect of intranasal obstruction on breathing during sleep. Chest. 1986; 90:324–329.

22. Metes A, Cole P, Hoffstein V, and Miljeteig H. Nasal airway dilation and obstructed breathing in sleep. Laryngoscope. 1992; 102:1053–1055.

23. Young T, Finn L, and Kim H. Chronic nasal congestion at night is a risk factor for snoring: in population-based cohort study. Arch Intern Med. 2001; 161:1514–1519.

24. Lenders H, Schaefer J, and Pirsig W. Turbinate hypertrophy in habitual snorers and patients with sleep apnea: findings of acoustic rhinometry. Laryngoscope. 1991; 101:614–618.

25. Silvioniemi P, Suonpaa J, Sipila J, et al. Sleep disorders in patients with severe nasal obstruction due to septal deviation. Acta Otolaryngol. 1997; 529:199–201.

26. Verse T, Pirsig W, and Kroker BA. Obstructive Schlafapnoe und polypsosis nasi. Laryngorhinootologie. 1998; 77:150–152.

27. Friedman M, Tanyeri H, Lim J, Landsberg R, et al. Effects of improved nasal breathing on obstructive sleep apnea. Otolaryngol Head Neck Surg. 2000; 122:71–74.

28. Kim ST, Choi JH, Jeon JG, et al. Polysomnographic effects of nasal surgery for snoring and obstructive sleep apnea. Acta Otolaryngol. 2004; 124:297–300.

29. Verse T, Maurer J, and Pirsig W. Effects of nasal surgery on sleep-related breathing disorders. Laryngoscope. 2002; 112:64–68.

30. Friedman M, Ibrahim H, and Joseph N. Staging of obstructive sleep apnea/hypopnea syndrome: a guide to appropriate treatment. Laryngoscope. 2004; 114(3):434–439.

31. Verse T, Kroker B, Pirsig W, et al. Tonsillectomy as a treatment of obstructive sleep apnea in adults with tonsillar hypertrophy. Laryngoscope. 2000; 110(9):1556–1559.

32. Guilleminuault C and Abad V. Obstructive sleep apnea. Curr Treat Options Neurol. 2004; 6(4):309–317.

33. Hall D, Littlefield P, Birkmire-Peters D, et al. Radiofrequency ablation versus electrocautery in tonsillectomy. Otolaryngol Head Neck Surg. 2004; 130(3):300–305.

34. Fischer Y, Kahn M, and Mann W. Multilevel temperature-controlled radiofrequency therapy of soft palate, base of tongue, and tonsils in adults with obstructive sleep apnea. Laryngoscope. 2003; 113(10):1786–1791.

35. Ikematsu T. Study of snoring, 4th report: therapy (in Japanese). Jpn Otol Rhinol Laryngol Soc. 1964; 64:434–435.

36. Fujita S, Conway W, Zorick F, et al. Surgical correction of anatomic abnormalities in obstructive sleep apnea syndrome: uvulopalatopharyngoplasty. Otolaryngol Head Neck Surg. 1981; 89(6):923–934.

37. Fairbanks DNF. Operative techniques of uvulopalatopharyngoplasty: operative techniques in otolaryngology. Head Neck Surg. 1991; 2:104–105.

38. Kezirian E, Weaver E, Yueh B, et al. Incidence of serious complications after uvulopalatopharyngoplasty. Laryngoscope. 2004; 114(3):450–453.

39. Senior B, Rosenthal L, Lumley A, et al. Effectiveness of uvulopalatopharyngoplasty in unselected patients for mild obstructive sleep apnea. Otolaryngol Head Neck Surg. 2000; 123(3):179–182.

40. Dickson RI and Blokmanis A. Treatment of obstructive sleep apnea by uvulopalatopharyngoplasty. Laryngoscope. 1987; 97:1054–1059.

41. Simmons FB, Guilleminault C, and Silvestri R. Snoring, and some obstructive sleep apnea, can be cured by oropharyngeal surgery. Arch Otolaryngol. 1983; 109:503–507.

42. Larsson LH, Carlsson-Nordlander B, and Svanborg E. Four-year follow-up after uvulopalatopharyngoplasty in 50 unselected patients with obstructive sleep apnea syndrome. Laryngoscope. 1994; 104:1362–1368.

43. Riley R, Powell N, and Guilleminault C. Obstructive sleep apnea syndrome: a review of 306 consecutively treated surgical patients. Otolaryngol Head Neck Surg. 1993; 108:117–125.

44. Sher A. Upper airway surgery for obstructive sleep apnea. Sleep Med Rev. 2002; 6:195–212.

45. Riley R, Guilleminault C, Powell N, et al. Palatopharyngoplasty failure, cephalometric roentgenograms, and obstructive sleep apnea. Otolaryngol Head Neck Surg. 1985; 93:240–244.

46. Bettega G, Pepin J, Veale D, et al. Obstructive sleep apnea syndrome: fifty-one consecutive patients treated by maxillfacial surgery. Am J Respir Crit Care Med. 2000; 162(2):641–649.

47. DeRowe A, Gunther E, Fibbi A, et al. Tonge-base suspension with a soft tissue-to-bone anchor for obstructive sleep apnea: preliminary clinical results of a new minimally invasive technique. Otolaryngol Head Neck Surg. 2000; 122:100–103.

48. Coleman J and Bick PA. Suspension sutures for the treatment of obstructive sleep apnea and snoring. Otolaryngol Clin North Am. 1999; 32:277–285.

49. Omur M, Ozturan D, Elez F, et al. Tongue base suspensión combined with UPPP in severe OSA patients. Otolaryngol Head Neck Surg. 2005; 133:218–223.

50. Miller F, Watson D, and Boseley M. The role of the Genial bone advancement trephine system in conjunction with uvulopalatopharyngoplasty in the multilevel management of obstructive sleep apnea. Otolaryngol Head Neck Surg. 2004; 13(1):73–79.

51. Mirza N and Lanza DC. The nasal airway and obstructed breathing during sleep. Otolaryngol Clin North Am. 1999; 32:243–262.

52. Wodson BT and Fujita S. Clinical experience with lingualplasty as part of the treatment of severe obstructive sleep apnea. Otolaryngol Head Neck Surg. 1992; 107:40–48.

53. Powell N, Riley R, Troell R, et al. Radiofrequency volumetric reduction of the tongue: a porcine pilot study for the treatment of obstructive sleep apnea syndrome. Chest. 1997; 111:1348–1355.

54. Back L, Tervahartiala P, Piilonen A, et al. Bipolar radiofrequency thermal ablation of the soft palate in habitual snorers without significant desaturations assessed by magnetic resonance imaging. Am J Resp Crit Care Med. 2002; 166(6):865–871.

55. Kania R, Schmitt E, Petelle B, et al. Radiofrequency soft palate procedure in snoring: influence of energy delivered. Otolaryngol Head Neck Surg. 2004; 130(1):67–72.

56. Powell N, Riley R, Troell R, et al. Radiofrequency volumetric tissue reduction of the palate in subjects with sleep-disordered breathing. Chest. 1998; 113(5):1163–1174.

57. Terris D, Coker J, Thomas A, et al. Preliminary findings from a prospective, randomized trial of two palatal operations for sleep-disordered breathing. Otolaryngol Head Neck Surg. 2002; 127(4):315–323.

58. Dattilo D and Drooger S. Outcome assessment of patients undergoing maxillofacial procedures for the treatment of sleep apnea: comparison of subjective and objective results. J Oral Maxillofac Surg. 2004; 62:164–168.

59. Powell NB, Riley RW, and Guilleminault C. Radiofrequency tongue base reduction in sleep disordered breathing: a pilot study. Otolaryngol Head Neck Surg. 1999; 120:656–664.

60. Steward D. Effectiveness of multilevel (tongue and palate) radiofrequency tissue ablation for patients with obstructive sleep apnea syndrome. Laryngoscope. 2004; 114(12):2073–2084.

61. Robinson S, Lewis R, Norton A, et al. Ultrasound-guided radiofrequency submucosal tongue-base excision for sleep apnea: a preliminary report. Clin Otolaryngol Allied Sci. 2003; 109:1901–1907.

62. Friedman M, Soans R, Gurpinar B, et al. Evaluation of submucosal minimally invasive lingual excision technique for treatment of obstructive sleep apnea/hypopnea syndrome. Otolaryngol Head Neck Surg. 2008; 139:378–384.

63. Riley R, Powell N, Guillemiault C, et al. Obstructive sleep apnea trends in therapy. West J Med. 1995; 162:143–148.

64. Sher A, Schechtman K, and Piccirillo J. An American Sleep Disorders Association review: the efficacy of surgical modifications of the upper airway in adults with obstructive sleep apnea syndrome. Sleep. 1996; 19:156–177.

65. Riley R, Powell N, and Guilleminault C. Obstructive sleep apnea and the hyoid: a revised surgical procedure. Otolaryngol Head Neck Surg. 1994; 111:717–721.

66. Verse T, Baisch A, and Hormann K. Multi-level surgery for obstructive sleep apnea. Preliminary objective results. Laryngorhinootologie. 2004; 83:516–522.

67. Bowden M, Kezirian E, Utley D, et al. Outcomes of hyoid suspension for the treatment of obstructive sleep apnea. Arch Otolaryngol Head Neck Surg. 2005; 131:440–445.

68. Waite PD and Shahidhar MS. Maxillomandibular advancement surgery: a cure for obstructive sleep apnea syndrome. Oral Maxillofac Surg Clin North Am. 1995; 7:327–344.

69. Prinsell JR. Maxillomandibular advancement surgery in a site-specific treatment approach for obstructive sleep apnea in fifty consecutive patients. Chest. 1999; 116:1519–1529.

70. Li K, Powell N, Riley R, et al. Long-term results of maxillomandibular advancement surgery. Sleep Breath. 2000; 4:137–139.

71. Petruson B. Snoring can be reduced when the nasal airflow is increased by the nasal dialtor Nozovent. Arch Otolaryngol head Neck Surg. 1990; 116:462–464.

72. Djupesland PG, Stakvedt O, and Borgersen A. Dichotomous physiological effects of nocturnal external nasal dilation in heavy snorers: the answer to a rhinologic controversy? Am J Rhinol. 2001; 15:95–103.

73. Gosepath J, Amedee R, Romanstschuk S, and Mann W. Breathe Right nasal strips and respiratory disturbance index in sleep related breathing disorders. Am J Rhinol. 1999; 13:385–389.

74. Liistro G, Rombaux P, Dury M, et al. Effects of breath right on snoring: a polysomnographic study. Respir Med. 1998; 92:1076–1078.

75. Schonhofer B, Franklin K, Brunig H, et al. Effect of nasal valve dilation on obstructive sleep apnea. Chest. 2000; 118:587–590.

# 11

# Oral appliance therapy for sleep-related breathing disorders

## CONCEPTUAL OVERVIEW

Oral appliance (OA) therapy has been used for the management of sleep-related breathing disorders (SRBD) since the early 1930s.[1] Subsequent investigations into the obstruction of the upper airway led to the study of OA therapy as a nonsurgical treatment option. These early research endeavors identified OA devices that were of two different designs: (1) mandibular repositioning appliance (MRA) that advanced the mandible in a protrusive position and (2) tongue-retaining device (TRD) that held the tongue in an advanced position. Both these OA designs demonstrated promise in reducing the upper airway obstruction.[2-4] Following these early discoveries, there has been a myriad of studies assessing the clinical efficacy and long-term use of OA therapy for the management of SRBD.

The first standards of practice guidelines relative to the use and effectiveness of OA therapy for obstructive sleep apnea (OSA) and snoring were published in 1995 by the American Academy of Sleep Medicine (AASM, formerly the American Sleep Disorders Association).[5] Case studies comprised the evidence on which those initial clinical guidelines were based. The AASM guidelines document noted that OA therapy can be considered as a first-line treatment option for the management of mild OSA and simple snoring and also as a second-line treatment option for moderate OSA after unsuccessful attempts with other treatment options. Following the publication of these guidelines, significant research-based findings pertaining to OA therapy have been published.[6]

In 2006, the AASM published two documents that further recognized OA therapy as a medical device option for the management of OSA and snoring: (1) an evidence-based review of literature regarding OA therapy in sleep medicine[6] and (2) a practice parameters update.[7] Scientific literature published since 1995 comprised the evidence on which the current practice parameters were based. The updated practice parameters indicate that OA therapy is now an option for patients with mild to moderate sleep apnea *and* who prefer this method of treatment as opposed to using continuous positive airway pressure (CPAP). In addition, OA therapy may be utilized in patients with severe sleep apnea who (1) are unable to tolerate CPAP, (2) have failed surgery, or (3) are primary (benign) snorers (i.e., snoring without apnea).

OAs have also been reviewed by the United States Food and Drug Administration (FDA), and OAs are regarded as class II medical devices.[8] The FDA document states that special controls apply to these devices, and they are deemed to be medical devices appropriate for the treatment of OSA. As such, OAs marketed to the public for the treatment/management of OSA and snoring are required to have a 510(k) or premarket notification clearance in order to be commercially available.

## HISTORY OF OAs

In the early part of the 1900s, the first OA that repositioned the mandible was used to address mandibular retrognathia.[9] Of interest, this particular device also had a positive secondary effect on the airway. In the 1950s, OAs were utilized mainly to stimulate growth of the mandible for correction of a malocclusion, and they were, for the most part, not recognized for their role in airway improvement during sleep.

In the 1960s and 1970s, research related to the impact of OAs on the growth of the mandible was increasing. During this time, the impact on the airway from OAs designed to reposition the mandible was also being investigated.[10] The research demonstrated the impact that airway compromise and obstruction had on growth of the mandible as well as the rest of the craniofacial complex. Accordingly, the resolution of airway compromise along with the resultant improved breathing had the potential to beneficially impact human growth and development.

The first available OA that was designed specifically for the management of SRBD was a TRD developed by a physician who was attempting to treat his own sleep breathing issues.[11, 12] Fabricated out of a flexible material with a bulb-like receptacle in the anterior portion, the TRD was intended to pull and maintain the tongue in a forward position during sleep so that the tongue would not collapse into the airway against the posterior pharyngeal wall, especially since there can be a tendency for the musculature to exhibit decreased muscle tone during sleep (Figures 11.1a–11.1c).

Other OA designs were introduced in the 1980s and 1990s, all of which were intended to reposition or advance the mandible to improve the upper

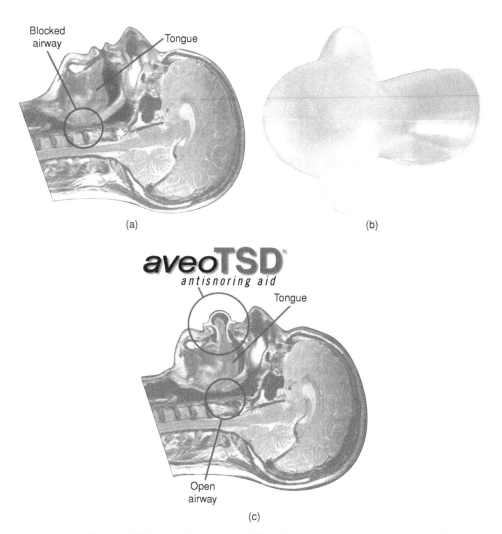

(a)

(b)

(c)

**Figure 11.1**   (a) Sagittal MRI of head: supine position demonstrating blocked airway from base of tongue impinging against posterior pharyngeal airway. (Courtesy of Innovative Health Technologies, 2009. Used with permission.) (b) Sample of a TRD: "aveoTSD". (Courtesy of Innovative Health Technologies, 2009. Used with permission.) (c) Sagittal MRI of head: supine position demonstrating an opened airway from the use of the "aveoTSD" to maintain an advanced position of the tongue. (Courtesy of Innovative Health Technologies, 2009. Used with permission.)

airway patency. All these OA designs were referred to as anterior repositioning or mandibular repositioning OAs, with the term MRA often used.

The devices that were introduced in the 1980s were mostly a one-piece design that joined the maxillary and mandibular acrylic components together, and they were referred to as monoblocs (Figures 11.2a and 11.2b). However, this particular design did not allow for any mandibular

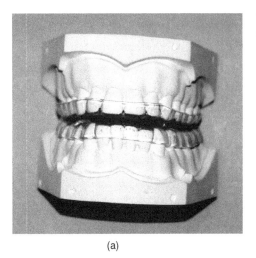
(a)

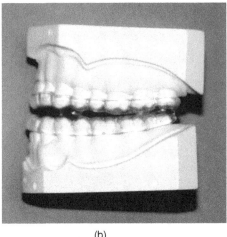
(b)

**Figure 11.2**    (a) Frontal view of monobloc type of MRA design. (b) Sagittal view of monobloc type of MRA design.

movement, such as the teeth grinding component of bruxism, and some patients reported discomfort with the masticatory muscles and/or temporomandibular joints (TMJs) after wearing this rigid type of design. In addition, if an alternative maxillomandibular relationship was deemed necessary for therapeutic or patient comfort purposes, it was not possible to modify the MRA without having to either (1) remake the entire OA or (2) separate the two components and reconnect them in a different maxillomandibular relationship with acrylic.

From the 1990s to the present time, most devices have been fabricated as separate maxillary and mandibular acrylic-type components that are joined together in a specific fashion that is unique to their respective manufacturer's mechanism, material, and purpose. Although the means by which the separate components are held together vary by manufacturer, the majority of them (1) account for bruxism by allowing for some degree of mandibular lateral excursions and (2) permit incremental anteroposterior adjustability (titration) for the dentist to easily modify the maxillomandibular relationship for optimum therapeutic effectiveness and patient comfort.

# TREATMENT PROTOCOL, OBJECTIVES, AND CONTRAINDICATIONS

Because snoring and OSA are regarded as medical conditions, the dentist and physician need to cooperate with each other regarding the pretreatment assessment and management plan for the patient. The AASM[6] and the American Academy of Dental Sleep Medicine[13] recommend similar treatment protocols for utilizing OA therapy in the management of OSA and snoring.

Both protocols outline the roles of the dentist and physician:

1.  Assessment by a sleep physician: (a) the dentist can refer the patient to the physician to diagnose the SRBD via an overnight sleep study, and then the patient returns to the dentist if OA therapy is medically indicated, or (b) the patient is initially referred to the dentist by the sleep physician if OA therapy is medically indicated via an overnight sleep study.
2.  The sleep physician provides the dentist with a written referral as well as copy of the diagnostic sleep study report.
3.  The dentist assesses if the patient is a candidate for OA therapy, and the patient is advised of the appropriate OA design(s) for that patient as well as of the fees. Examples of OA designs should be shown to the patient, and a rationale for the appropriate OA design should be explained to the patient and documented in the patient record.
4.  An informed consent about the risks and benefits of OA therapy for SRBD is obtained from the patient and documented in the patient record.
5.  OA therapy is initiated by the dentist, which includes titration appointments as needed to obtain optimum effectiveness relative to the patient's initial symptoms.
6.  Subsequent to the titration period, the patient is referred back to the sleep physician for medical assessment by the sleep physician relative to the OA's therapy effectiveness.
7.  The final resolution of SRBD is determined by the sleep physician, typically with an overnight sleep study. If the initial medical diagnosis was primary snoring, then the dentist may complete OA therapy without the referral back to the sleep physician.
8.  If medical assessment by the sleep physician demonstrates continued SRBD, then the dentist may need to consider additional titration of the MRA. The sleep physician may also recommend alternative treatment options, if appropriate.
9.  An annual dental follow-up assessment is recommended for all OSA or snoring patients who have pursued OA therapy, especially since SRBD can have the tendency to worsen over time.

The AASM documents relative to its practice parameters and evidence-based review of literature lay the scientific foundation for the AASM's recommendations about the use of OA therapy for the management of OSA or snoring.[6,7] The AASM defined the three levels of recommendations used in those documents as follows:

●   *Standard*: "This is a generally accepted patient-care strategy, which reflects a high degree of clinical certainty."

- *Guideline*: "This is a patient-care strategy, which reflects a moderate degree of clinical certainty."
- *Option*: "This is a patient-care strategy, which reflects uncertain clinical use."

When considering the recommendations in the practice parameters, these definitions will serve as references for the dentist when engaging in the management of patients with OSA and/or snoring.

## Assessment prior to initiation of treatment

Regarding assessment and diagnosis of SRBD relative to OA therapy, the AASM's practice parameters made the following recommendation:[7]

> The presence or absence of OSA must be determined before initiating treatment with oral appliances to identify those patients at risk due to complications of sleep apnea and to provide a baseline to establish the effectiveness of subsequent treatment. Detailed diagnostic criteria for OSA are available and include clinical signs, symptoms and the findings identified by polysomnography. The severity of sleep related respiratory problems must be established in order to make an appropriate treatment decision. (Standard)

## Treatment objectives

Once the pretreatment assessment and diagnosis have been accomplished and OA therapy has been established as a treatment option for the SRBD patient, then the following treatment objectives for OA therapy in the management of SRBD, specifically OSA and snoring, are recommended per the AASM practice parameters:[7]

- "For patients with primary snoring without features of OSA or upper-airway resistance syndrome, the treatment objective is to reduce the snoring to a subjectively acceptable level. (Standard)"
- "For patients with OSA, the desired outcome of treatment includes the resolution of the clinical signs and symptoms of OSA and the normalization of the apnea-hypopnea index and oxyhemoglobin saturation. (Standard)"
- "Oral appliances are appropriate for use in patients with primary snoring who do not respond to or are not appropriate candidates for treatment with behavioral measures such as weight loss or sleep-position change. (Guideline)"
- "Although not as efficacious as CPAP, oral appliances are indicated for use in patients with mild to moderate OSA who prefer OAs to CPAP, or who do not respond to CPAP, are not appropriate candidates for CPAP, or who fail treatment attempts with CPAP or treatment

with behavioral measures such as weight loss or sleep-position change. (Guideline)"

- "Patients with severe OSA should have an initial trial of nasal CPAP because greater effectiveness has been shown with this intervention than with the use of oral appliances. Upper airway surgery (including tonsillectomy and adenoidectomy, craniofacial operations and tracheostomy) may also supersede use of oral appliances in patients for whom these operations are predicted to be highly effective in treating sleep apnea. (Guideline)"

## Dental contraindications

The following dental contraindications for OA therapy in the management of SRBD, specifically OSA and snoring, are identified per the AASM evidence-based review of literature:[6]

- "Patients need to have an adequate number of healthy teeth (not compromised by periodontal disease) in the upper and lower dental arch to use an MRA."
- "The patient should have the ability to protrude the mandible forward and open the jaw widely without significant limitation in order to be fitted with an MRA."
- "Moderate to severe TMJ problems or an inadequate protrusive ability may be contraindications to OA therapy—mild TMJ problems may be lessened by the forward jaw position."
- "Significant bruxism may be a contraindication to OA therapy."
- "Patients with full dentures are generally unable to use an MRA but some of these patients may be treated with a TD" (tongue device).

Table 11.1 summarizes the indications and contraindications for OA therapy in the management of SRBD, specifically OSA and snoring.

Even though the presence of severe temporomandibular disorders (TMD) may be overstated, the dentist needs to (1) recognize any preexisting TMD prior to the initiation of OA therapy for SRBD and (2) discern whether the TMD may need to be addressed accordingly. In many instances, the TMD is not an intracapsular disorder of the TMJ itself, but rather more of a disorder involving the soft tissue components of the TMJ and/or the musculature of the head and neck.

Frequently, the masticatory and cervical muscles are tender to palpation, and they may have ability to refer pain to the area of the TMJ (Table 11.2).[14] The ability for the musculature to refer pain to a location remote from the trigger points of the involved musculature is known as myofascial pain. Because the pain referral is from soft tissue, it typically can be relieved by exercise, physical medicine, and the use of muscle relaxation medications. In addition, the presence of sleep bruxism needs to be assessed since

**Table 11.1** Indications and contraindications for oral appliance therapy.

| Indications | Contraindications |
|---|---|
| Treatment of snoring alone (benign snoring) | Poor dental status |
| Patient with mild to moderate obstructive sleep apnea who *prefers* oral appliance over continuous positive airway pressure (CPAP) or did not respond to CPAP | Inadequate healthy teeth |
| Patient with severe sleep apnea who either failed CPAP or was intolerant to it | Active periodontal disease |
|  | Inadequate mandibular function or limited range of motion |
|  | Severe temporomandibular disorders |

*Source:* Adapted from Kushida CA, Morgenthaler TI, Littner MR, et al. Practice parameters for the treatment of snoring and obstructive sleep apnea with oral appliances: an update for 2005. Sleep. 2006; 29(2):240–262.

**Table 11.2** Myofascial pain and trigger point referral for the most common muscles of the jaw and neck associated with oral appliance therapy.

| Muscle | Common site for referral |
|---|---|
| Temporalis | Forehead and over the eyes |
|  | Maxillary teeth (anterior portion to the anterior teeth, middle portion to the bicuspids, posterior portion to the molars) |
| Masseter | Ear and around the temporomandibular joint (TMJ) area |
|  | Supraorbital region |
|  | Mandibular posterior teeth |
| Lateral pterygoid | TMJ area |
|  | Mid-face and infraorbital area |
| Medial pterygoid | TMJ and surrounding area |
|  | Posterior face and mandible |
| Sternocleidomastoid | Face, supraorbital, back and top of the head, under the mandible |
|  | Ear, behind the ear, forehead (only muscle that will refer across the midline to the other side of the forehead) |
| Diagatrics | Anterior teeth |
|  | Neck, under the mandible at the posterior aspect (may feel like a sore throat) |
| Posterior cervicals | Face and TMJ area |
|  | Forehead and the temples |
|  | Back of the head |

*Source:* Adapted from Travell JG and Simons DG. Myofascial Pain and Dysfunction: The Trigger Point Manual. Baltimore: Williams & Wilkins. 1983.

it can be associated with snoring and OSA, and it may be a precipitating mechanism.[15,16]

## FUNCTION OF MRA THERAPY

For the management of OSA and snoring, the basic function of OA therapy with an MRA design is to reposition the mandible in an increased vertical or open position as well as in an advanced or protrusive position relative to the maxilla. The basic function of a TRD design is to hold the tongue in a more forward position. Although the exact mechanism of the OA on the airway is not fully understood, it is believed that OA therapy improves the patency of the upper airway by increasing the pharyngeal volume or size and/or reducing the collapsibility of the airway through muscle tone improvement.

The upper airway of OSA patients is more narrowed during sleep than those who do not have OSA.[17] Studies have shown that anterior repositioning of the mandible and tongue increases the size and volume of the upper airway, typically in the retropalatal and retroglossal areas.[18–24] Not all studies, though, demonstrate such airway size increase. One study found that there was no change in the airway size with mandibular advancement.[25] Lending to the suggestion that increasing the airway size beneficially affects the severity of OSA are the studies that reflect a reduced apnea–hypopnea index (AHI) with increased mandibular advancement.[26–29]

Repositioning the mandible also impacts the muscles that support the pharyngeal airway and comprise the tongue. The action of mandibular repositioning may do the following: (1) prevent the tongue from collapsing posteriorly into the oropharyngeal area and (2) stabilize the musculature that supports the airway. A study demonstrated that improvement in the airway is impacted by the palatoglossus muscle on the tongue base when accompanied by mandibular opening.[30]

The musculature that is related to the tongue and the pharynx may also be beneficially affected by mandibular repositioning. With the mandible advanced, the musculature of the pharynx and the tongue are stabilized, thus preventing these structures from collapsing, narrowing, and obstructing the pharynx during snoring or OSA. Studies on mandibular and tongue advancement with OA therapy found increased muscle tone of the upper airway and decreased genioglossus muscle tone.[31,32]

In addition, the repositioning of the mandible also positively impacts the velopharyngeal area and thereby improves the patient's ability to nose breath.[33] It is believed that the MRA's impact on the palatopharyngeus creates an increased amount of tension on the soft palate, and the repositioning moves the tongue base forward and away from the inferior surface of the soft palate, resulting in increased patency of the nasopharynx for improved breathing (Figures 11.3–11.6).

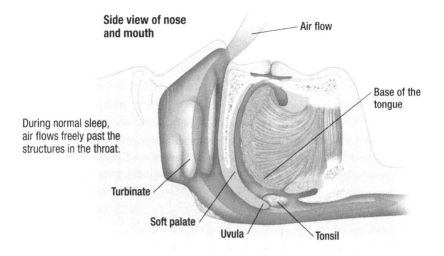

**Figure 11.3**    Normal sagittal view of the upper airway. (© Krames Medical Publishing, 2009. Used with permission.)

## DESIGN CHARACTERISTICS OF MRAs

For MRAs to be optimally effective and reduce the impact of side effects, there are several design characteristics that should be considered when selecting an MRA design. The selection should be based on (1) specific and related medical and dental conditions of the patient, (2) patient preference,

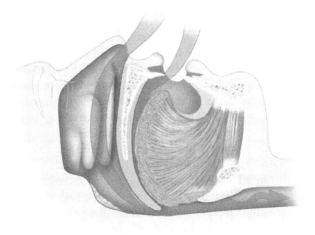

**Figure 11.4**    Sagittal view of partially blocked upper airway. (© Krames Medical Publishing, 2009. Used with permission.)

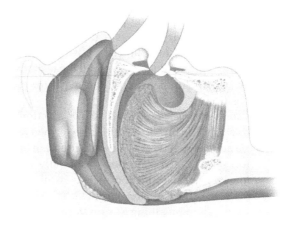

**Figure 11.5**  Sagittal view of completely blocked upper airway. (© Krames Medical Publishing, 2009. Used with permission.)

and knowledge, experience, and preferences of the dentist providing the service.

The following are suggested characteristics of MRAs for optimum effect in the management of OSA and snoring:

- *Adjustable:* It (1) is easily adjusted to accommodate changes in the dental status, (2) can be modified to address a new dental restoration, and (3) can be relined to improve retention or the fit.

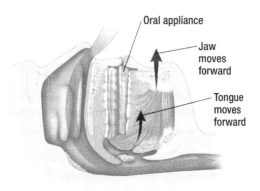

Oral appliance

Jaw
moves
forward

Tongue
moves
forward

Moving the jaw and tongue forward with an
oral appliance can open the airway to reduce
sleep apnea.

**Figure 11.6**  Sagittal view of an opened airway from the use of an OA. (© Krames Medical Publishing, 2009. Used with permission.)

- *Posterior support:* It (1) addresses sleep bruxism as well as SRBD and (2) provides adequate support for the TMJs.
- *Titration:* It incorporates a mechanism that allows incremental positional changes (e.g., anterior, posterior, vertical).
- *Full coverage of teeth:* It covers all the teeth to prevent tooth movement or unwanted supereruption, and maintains the teeth in the pretreatment position.
- *Mandibular mobility:* It (1) allows freedom of mandibular movement during sleep bruxism that is also termed as rhythmic masticatory muscle activity, which is commonly found in all patients; (2) improves comfort of the OA during sleep, especially with sleep bruxism; and (3) allows for normal function such as swallowing and licking the lips.
- *Lip seal and patent nasal airway:* It (1) allows for comfortable lip seal to limit mouth breathing during sleep and (2) improves blood oxygen saturation levels via an open nasal airway, otherwise adjunctive treatment of the nasal airway may be required.
- *Maximum tongue space:* It affords maximum space for the tongue to prevent further collapse of the tongue into the pharyngeal airway space, especially since encroachment of the OA into the tongue space may cause the tongue to be in a more posterior position in the mouth.

## EFFECTIVENESS OF OAs

There are a number of studies and literature reviews that have evaluated OAs and their effectiveness, including the AASM evidence-based review of literature which included objective sleep data before and after OA therapy.[6] Another literature review document also summarized in 2007 many of the studies published on OAs relative to their effectiveness for the management of SRBD.[34] Although the data in these documents support the use of OAs, it continues to be difficult to predict an outcome with OA therapy for any specific SRBD patient. Other than an objective sleep study that includes a polysomnogram, the currently accepted means by which OA effectiveness can be reliably documented through self-reports is with the use of the Epworth Sleepiness Scale (ESS). It has been shown that the ESS score was improved in OA users from 11.2 to 7.8,[34] and other self-report assessments also demonstrated significant reductions in ESS scores regarding the efficacy of OA therapy.[27,35–37]

When using respiratory sleep data to assess the affect of OA therapy on severity of respiratory disturbances for individuals with OSA, the definition of success varied among the studies considered in the AASM review of literature: "the most stringent definition of success was a reduction to less than five respiratory events per hour of sleep while the most liberal definition was a reduction of 50% or more from the baseline AHI."[6]

OAs have also been found to be effective in the improvement of cardiovascular disease. Three studies documented improvement in blood pressure measurements with the use of OA therapy.[35,38,39] One study found that in 161 patients who used an OA for 60 days, the improvement in the blood pressure went from 132.0/82.1 to 127.5/79.2. Another study indicated that the improvement in blood pressure was equivalent to that found with the use of CPAP therapy.

A study that evaluated oxidative stress after 1 year with the use of an OA demonstrated improvement in the AHI, ESS, and endothelial function.[40] Although the apneic events were not totally eliminated, there was improvement that offered encouragement for these conditions in the future.

Effectiveness of OA therapy has also been evaluated relative to other therapies, such as CPAP and surgery, as well as comparison among different OA designs.

## Comparison of OAs with CPAP

There are several crossover studies that have compared MRA therapy with CPAP.[37,41–45] The findings in each of the studies confirmed that CPAP was more efficacious in reducing the AHI to normal levels as well as controlling snoring in almost all patients, whereas OA therapy was able to do the same in about two-thirds of the patients. However, these studies also indicated that OA therapy was the preferred method of treatment. In addition, the use of an OA demonstrated better compliance when compared to CPAP. One such study found that in 41 patients who had utilized both an OA and CPAP, 71% preferred the OA.[46]

## Comparison of OAs with surgery

For comparison of OA therapy and upper airway surgery, there has been one randomized parallel study,[47] several related reports,[48–51] and two reviews of literature documents.[6,34] Results found that after 1 year, 51% of the uvulopalatopharyngoplasty (UPPP) surgery patients had an AHI less than 10 compared to 78% of the OA patients. At the 4-year interval, 3% of the UPPP surgery patients and 63% of the OA group had an AHI less than 10.

The one surgery that appears to have the best prognosis as compared to OAs is maxillomandibular advancement surgery.[52] In one study, 4 patients out of a total of 43 with an OA had an initial AHI of 50 that decreased to 12, and the AHI for the surgery group was reduced to 2.

# FABRICATION AND DELIVERY OF THE OA

The following recommendation for the dental management, including the fitting of an OA, for patients with OSA is provided by the AASM practice parameters for OAs and was based on committee consensus:[6]

- "Oral appliances should be fitted by qualified dental personnel who are trained and experienced in the overall care of oral health, the temporomandibular joint, dental occlusion and associated oral structures. Dental management of patients with OAs should be overseen by practitioners who have undertaken serious training in sleep medicine and/or sleep related breathing disorders with focused emphasis on the proper protocol for diagnosis, treatment, and follow up. (Option)"

## Informed consent

There are a number of informed consent examples available for the use of OA therapy for the management of SRBD. Some of the OA manufacturers have ones that are unique to their specific device. The American Academy of Dental Sleep Medicine provides one that is available only to their members and it is generalized for all OAs.

Regardless of which one is selected or developed, it is advisable for the dentist to contact his or her malpractice insurance carrier or an attorney regarding specific content of the consent form. The major factors of concern are to be certain that the patient is advised of the need for ongoing follow-up care, the side effect potentials, and the use and care of the OA. It is also important that the patients have had any questions or concerns answered, and that this communication has been documented in the patient record. The follow-up visits should also be documented in detail, particularly relative to any side effects as well as improvement in the patient's symptoms and sleep quality.

## Making impressions

The actual fabrication of the OA starts with the process of obtaining impressions of the patient's maxillary and mandibular teeth and related structures, which are subsequently poured into stone casts. The impression material should be stable and provide a detailed representation of the teeth and surrounding structures. Material selected for the impressions can be (1) a quality alginate, (2) one of the products on the market that is designed as an alginate substitute, or (3) a polyvinylsiloxane. The advantage of alginate substitute and polyvinylsiloxane materials is the allowance for the dentist to do multiple pours of the impression, which affords the option of maintaining a pretreatment cast for future reference. Retaining duplicates of the master casts as part of the record can be helpful in the event that there are concerns regarding tooth movement or changes in the maxillomandibular relationship. In addition, these retained casts may be needed for future use in the event that repairs to the OA are needed because of fracture or breakage.

The mandibular impression should provide adequate detail of the teeth and all the lingual anatomy with appropriate extension into these areas. If there are mandibular lingual tori present, these should be captured in the impression so that the master cast has sufficient detail for the dental laboratory to provide relief around them or to design the OA's mandibular component to circumnavigate the tori.

The maxillary impression should also have adequate detail of the teeth and the hard palatal area. Depending on the OA design, it may or may not be necessary for the entire hard palate to be captured in the impression. If the anteroposterior adjustment (titration) mechanism is going to be located in the palatal vault region, then it would be necessary to capture that palatal aspect in the impression. If such mechanism design is not going to be employed in that palatal region, then it would not be as necessary to capture the complete palatal area since the hard palate will not be totally covered by the OA's maxillary component. For some patients, covering the entire hard palate has the potential of interfering with proper tongue space and position during function (e.g., swallowing).

After the impressions are obtained, they need to be poured in a relatively hard stone, usually the typical die stone used for fixed prosthodontics. These casts along with the interocclusal record (IR) will be sent to the dental laboratory for the fabrication of the appliance.

If there is any concern about the impressions for the fabrication of the OA or the cast that is needed, it is always best to contact the dental laboratory that will be fabricating the appliance for clarification and/or their specifications per the OA design.

## Interocclusal record

The IR, or bite registration, is typically established by the dentist at the same appointment as when the final impressions are obtained. The IR allows the dentist to determine the maxillomandibular relationship, or the therapeutic window, at which he or she will begin OA therapy for the SRBD patient. Generally, the therapeutic window is the three-dimensional anteroposterior and vertical positioning of the mandible relative to the maxilla that addresses the OSA and/or snoring.

If the dentist elects to employ an OA design that has a titration mechanism connecting the maxillary and mandibular components of the OA, then he or she has the ability to make incremental adjustments of that maxillomandibular relationship to potentially (1) modify the effectiveness of the OA regarding the OSA and/or snoring and (2) assist the patient's masticatory muscles and TMJs to slowly adapt to the optimum position in that three-dimensional therapeutic window.

A study assessed two OA designs and the patient's AHI responses to each design.[53] One of the designs repositioned the mandible anteriorly, and the other design was a placebo with no mandibular repositioning. The repositioning OA reduced the AHI, whereas there was no AHI improvement with the other OA design. Two prior studies and three subsequent studies reflected similar findings.[27,54–57] One of the studies used the same OA design, but compared AHI responses in two groups of patients relative to different amounts of mandibular advancement.[27] When comparing the two groups of 50 or 75% of the maximum distance that the patient could protrude, there was a reduction to <10 AHI in 31 and 52% of the patients, respectively.

The collective findings of these studies appear to indicate that greater degrees of mandibular advancement would result in greater reductions in AHI scores. As such, the therapeutic window for making the IR is typically in the 50–75% range of maximum mandibular protrusion.

Relative to the vertical opening component of the three-dimensional therapeutic window, studies have evaluated this component relative to OA effectiveness, but with mixed results (www.accessdata.fda.gov/scripts/cdrh/cfdocs/cfPMN/pmn.cfm).[22,42] Although this vertical component needs further investigation, the typical vertical opening of the IR can range from 2 to 10 or more millimeters, depending on the uniqueness of each individual patient case.

In addition, the IR fabrication technique and specifications may be available from the dental laboratory or the manufacturer for a specific OA design, and the dentist will need to use his or her best assessment when taking into account the patient's particular clinical case.

Table 11.3 outlines factors to consider when making the IR, and the following goals are associated with its use:

1.  Be able to maintain a lip seal with the OA seated on the dentition, which will foster nasal breathing during sleep.
2.  Provide the least amount of strain on the masticatory musculature with the use of the OA.
3.  Focus on the combined approach of mandibular advancement and vertical opening: (a) for optimum effectiveness of the OA and (b) to lessen the possibility of occlusal changes with the use of an OA.

Making the IR can be accomplished in a variety of ways. The use of a device called the George Gauge© has been a very standard technique (Figure 11.7).

The George Gauge© is composed of a handle to which a bite fork component is attached. The handle portion is designed to (1) hold the bite fork and (2) allow for the determination of the amount of advancement that is desired by virtue of a sliding scale on the one side. On the opposite side, there is the ability to adjust the thickness of that portion that fits over the mandibular anterior teeth by loosening the setscrew and sliding the lingual portion forward or backward. This allows for variations in the size of the teeth as well as accommodates for crowding or rotations of the anterior teeth. The device also has a midline mark indicator for the maxillary teeth that can be used as a reference point.

The bite fork component is designed such that two different vertical measurements can be obtained, 2 mm or 5 mm, in the interincisal area. The 5 mm bite fork is typically more frequently used as it allows for interarch spacing in the posterior areas necessary for most OA designs. If additional vertical spacing is desired, the incisal notch of the maxillary portion of the

**Table 11.3** Proposed interocclusal record for oral appliances: initial starting position for mandibular repositioning appliance design.

| | |
|---|---|
| Vertical | Start at between 5 and 7 mm interincisally (Edge to edge)<br>Take into consideration<br>    Maintain a lip seal<br>    Able to nose breathe<br>    Inability to voluntarily snore<br>    Subjective improvement in airway |
| Advancement of mandible based on relationship of incisors and angles classification | Class I (full dentition) |
| | Incisors at edge to edge<br>Class I division 2<br>    Advanced 2–3 mm past edge to edge<br>Class I (previous bicuspid extraction)<br>    Advanced 1–4 mm past edge to edge<br>Class II division 1 to <5 mm overjet<br>    Advanced up to 5 mm—not beyond edge to edge<br>Class II division 1 to >5 mm overjet<br>    Advance up to 5 mm—not beyond<br>    Titrate advancement over time as deemed necessary<br>Class II division 2<br>    Advance 2–4 mm beyond edge to edge<br>Class III—prognathic mandible<br>    Minimal to no advancement<br>    Focus on vertical<br>Class III—retrognathic maxilla<br>    (Pseudo class III) Minimal advancement (1–3 mm) |

*Special Considerations:* In class III and more severe class II patients, a cephalometric radiograph should be done to evaluate the skeletal development of the patient.

bite fork can be modified by the addition of either a self-curing or light-curing acrylic. Once the proper bite fork has been selected, the amount of vertical should be verified with some type of measurement device such as a Boley gauge (Figure 11.8).

Occasionally, the groove of the bite fork that accommodates the maxillary teeth will need to be modified because of anatomical variation or crowding. The lingual portion of the groove is often adjusted or modified so that the bite fork is stable when seated on the anterior dentition.

## Delivery of the mandibular repositioning appliance

Delivery, or fitting, of the MRA for SRBD is similar to any other type of OA, although there may be adjustments and considerations unique to the

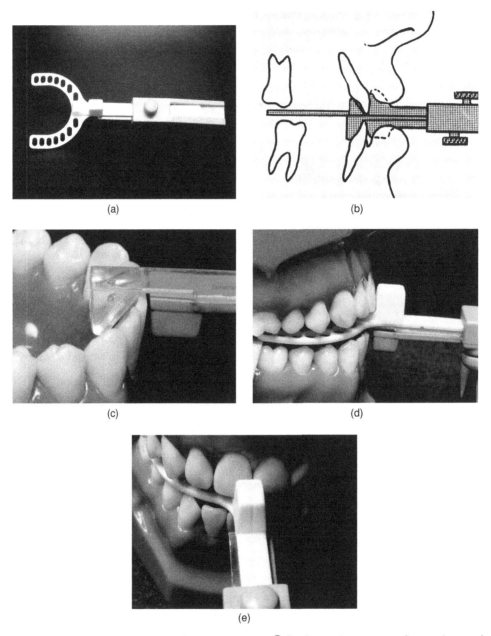

**Figure 11.7** (a) The George Gauge© for the IR. (b) Diagram of sagittal view of George Gauge© seated intraorally for making the IR. (c) Mandibular anterior clamp of George Gauge© adjusted to the lingual of the teeth for positioning of the anterior notch on the mandibular incisor teeth. (d) Sagittal view of George Gauge© in place ready for the IR material. (e) Frontal view of George Gauge© in place ready for the IR material.

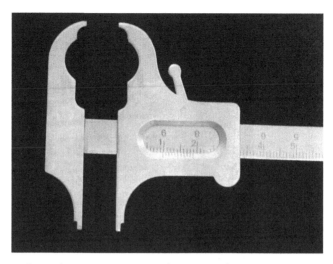

**Figure 11.8**    Boley gauge to assist in determining the optimum amount of vertical opening for the IR.

specific OA design being utilized. The major factors involved with the delivery of the MRA are the following:

*Optimum fit:* The device should be snug with adequate retention and should not cause discomfort to any of the teeth or to the masticatory musculature. It may initially feel tight to the patient because of the retention components of the OA, and there also may be masticatory muscle strain because of the mandibular advancement. If this is the case, the patient should be scheduled for a follow-up visit within a week after the delivery. At this time, the position of the mandible should be verified in accordance with the predetermined position that was established at the time of the IR.

*Adjustment of the OA's occlusal tables:* Many OAs have contact between the maxillary and mandibular components (posterior occlusion). This will need to be balanced and adjusted at the delivery appointment for comfort.

*Verify a lip seal:* Because a lip seal is optimum, this should be determined at this time. If the lip seal appears strained, possibly the vertical will need to be reduced at this time.

*Determine the ability to nose breathe:* Determine if the patient has the ability to adequately nose breath. If this appears to be a problem and the lip seal is adequate, then oftentimes the use of nasal strips may be helpful initially along with the use of nasal irrigation with a saline solution (Figure 11.9). One product that is very popular with physicians and is easy to use is the Neil Med Sinus rinse. It is a combine saline and sodium bicarbonate mixture that is prepackaged and is mixed with water.

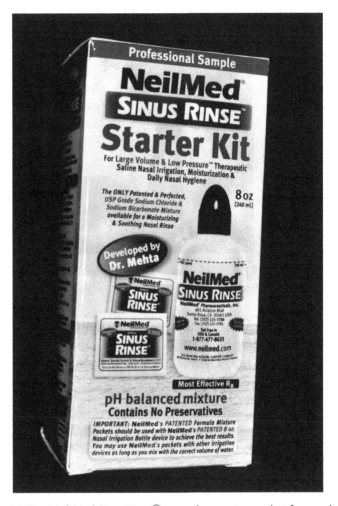

**Figure 11.9**    Neil Med Sinus Rinse©: over the counter product for nasal airway irrigation.

At this visit, the patient will need to be instructed in the proper use (removal and insertion), care, and the possible adverse effects associated with the use of an OA that repositions the mandible. Some of the manufacturers may have preprinted instructions that are available that can be given to patients when the appliance is delivered.

## Follow-up care

Follow-up care visits should be for the purpose of monitoring the outcome of the OA therapy. The frequency of these visits is determined by the progress that the patient makes with the OA, but the first follow-up visit is oftentimes within 2 weeks following the delivery of the OA. Oftentimes a patient will be appointed 4–6 times after the OA has been delivered over a 6-month time period, after which the patient will usually be aware of an improvement in their sleep as well as a decrease in the initial symptoms.

At each follow-up visit, the following may be addressed:

*Adjust the OA*: At these visits the overall fit, retention, posterior bite relationship, and comfort of the OA should be reviewed. Any needed adjustments should be made at this time and will be reviewed at a future follow-up visit.

*Assess the symptoms*: The original symptoms can be reviewed to determine if there is improvement. One of the key elements of major concern is snoring, an indicator that an adequate patent airway may not yet be achieved.

*Look for side effects*: At each follow-up visit, adverse outcomes of OA use should be evaluated, which includes maxillomandibular changes, tooth movement, masticatory muscle pain, and TMD-related findings. If there are any changes, then they need to be addressed immediately.

*Review the plan*: It is important to address the plan for the future. Because the patient has been sleep-deprived, they may not remember all the information related to the treatment from the previous visits.

## Testing for efficacy

The AASM practice parameters for OA therapy of OSA and snoring state the following relative to follow-up sleep testing:[7]

- "Follow-up sleep testing is not indicated for patients with primary snoring. (Guideline)
- To ensure satisfactory therapeutic benefit from OAs, patients with OSA should undergo polysomnography or an attended cardiorespiratory (Type 3) sleep study with the oral appliance in place after final adjustments of fit have been performed. (Guideline)
- Patients with OSA who are treated with oral appliances should return for follow-up visits with the dental specialist. Once optimal fit is obtained and efficacy shown, dental specialist follow-up at every 6 months is recommended for the first year, and at least annually thereafter. The purpose of the follow-up is to monitor patient adherence, evaluate device deterioration or maladjustment, evaluate the health of the oral structures and integrity of the occlusion, and assess the patient for signs and symptoms of worsening OSA. Intolerance and improper use of the device are potential problems for patients using oral appliances, which require patient effort to use properly. Oral appliances may aggravate temporomandibular joint disease and may cause dental misalignment and discomfort that are unique to each device. In addition,

oral appliances can be rendered ineffective by patient alteration of the device. (Option)

- Patients with OSA who are treated with oral appliances should return for periodic follow-up visits with the referring clinician. The purpose of the follow-up is to assess the patient for signs and symptoms of worsening OSA. Close communication with the dental specialist is most conducive to good patient care. An objective reevaluation of respiration during sleep is indicated if signs or symptoms of OSA worsen or reoccur. (Option)"

While the management of OSA with OA therapy is the dentist's role in the overall treatment of a medical condition, the ultimate responsibility for the SRBD patient belongs to the physician. This is particularly important to recognize given the large number of health-related consequences associated with sleep apnea.

Once the OA appears to have achieved an optimum result, follow-up testing is important to document. The follow-up testing can be accomplished in a variety of ways depending on the comfort level of the dentist providing the service. There are two major areas where improvement is best determined, neurocognitively and cardiovascularly. The neurocognitive improvement may be assessed with the ESS as well as subjective reports relative to the patient's mood and memory.

The ESS should be repeated periodically throughout the OA therapy period. If it was used prior to initiating the treatment, then this will help to determine if the patient's tendency to be drowsy during the day has improved. This is always a significant improvement particularly since being sleepy and/or tired are often associated with sleep apnea.

Improvement in mood and memory indicates improvement in brain function associated with improved sleep and possibly increased oxygen saturation levels. Although these parameters are subjectively reported by the patient and/or significant other, at least this information can be compared both pre- and post-OA therapy.

Improvement in the cardiovascular status of the patient may best be determined by obtaining the patient's blood pressure since it has been shown that OAs can improve the patient's blood pressure.

At this time, the use of portable monitoring devices for home sleep studies to determine the efficacy of the OA therapy may be utilized. There are many ambulatory devices available, and both the option of using this device to test the OA as well as which specific one to use has to be determined by the individual practitioner. The use of such devices should be considered in light of the comfort level of the dentist as well as their understanding of the specific recommendations for their use.

One place where such devices may have a role is in the initial phase of the treatment as a means of determining the performance level of the OA. A clinical guidelines paper published in 2007 indicates that the use of a Type 3 device that measures 4–7 channels of data is a valid indication for evaluating the response to non-CPAP treatment such as an OA.[58] This Type 3 device would allow for objective testing of the OA to determine if further adjustment or modification of the OA is warranted prior to referring the patient for a sleep study with the OA. At all times, the data from this testing should be shared with the sleep specialist and the patient's physician. In no way should the use of the portable monitoring devices be used to determine if the patient is at risk for OSA prior to them having a formal sleep study and diagnosis by the physician. This would most likely be viewed as practicing medicine without a license and is not within the scope of the practice of dentistry.

On the basis of the AASM practice parameters on OAs, the current recommendation is for the patient to have a formal overnight sleep study once the OA has been adjusted, titrated, and modified to the point of delivering an optimum outcome. Because a satisfactory, efficient, and cost-effective method of titrating an OA during the sleep study has not been developed as has been done for positive airway pressure (PAP), the overnight sleep study with the OA in place is the best way to test for the efficacy of the device.

# SIDE EFFECTS AND THEIR MANAGEMENT

Side effects with the use of OAs that reposition the mandible can be a concern. The overall long-term side effects are not well known. In many cases, patients will continue to use the OA despite the side effects as long as they are experiencing a positive result and outcome. The main reason that people stop using the OA is related to a lack of effective outcome. Compliance with the use of an OA is related to the perceived benefit despite the side effects. In one study it was found that compliance ranged from 48 to 84% after 2 years of use.[59]

The most common side effects or adverse outcomes and means by which they can be addressed are the following.

## Excessive salivation

This is more prevalent at the onset of treatment and usually subsides with the continued use of the OA.

*Intervention:* If this persists, then it may indicate that there is mouth breathing as a result of inadequate lip seal or restricted nasal airway or both. Patients who were chronic mouth breathers prior to receiving the OA may have the most difficulty. If the nasal airway is open, then the adjunctive use of a chin-up strip may be helpful to correct this issue.

## Face, muscle, and TMJ discomfort

This is most likely associated with the strain on the masticatory musculature associated with mandibular repositioning, which usually occurs in the

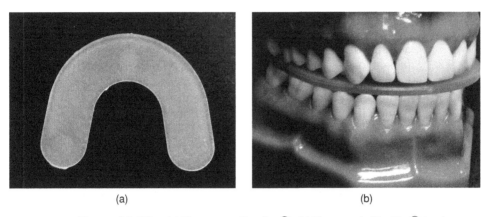

(a)                                                                    (b)

**Figure 11.10**    (a) Therapeutic Bite Rim©. (b) Therapeutic Bite Rim© in place.

early stages of OA therapy and typically resolves over time with continued use of the OA. Regarding any concern that OAs may cause a TMJ problem, this has not been found to be the case. In one study after a full year of OA therapy, the development of TMD was not found to be present and there were no morphologic changes involving the joints.[26]

*Intervention:* At times, intervention is needed to resolve these issues, but they can usually be managed with mandibular range of motion exercises. One such exercise involves the use of a therapeutic bite rim (Figures 11.10a and 11.10b).

The patient places the rim between the maxillary and mandibular teeth and subsequently slides the mandible anteriorly and posteriorly up to ten times after removing the OA. Also, the application of moist heat to the masseter areas while doing the exercises can be helpful. Sometimes a short course of muscle relaxation medications, such as Flexeril, Skelaxin, or a similar pharmaceutic, may help when taken prior to initiating sleep. In some situations, referring the patient for physical therapy may also be indicated if the problem persists.

## Maxillomandibular relationship or occlusal changes

One of the areas of major concern is a change in the maxillomandibular relationship or occlusion associated with the repositioning of the mandible for upwards of 6–8 hours a day. These changes may last for up to 30 minutes or longer after discontinuing the use of the OA.

*Intervention:* The use of the therapeutic bite rim can be helpful. In rare situations, the use of the OA has to be discontinued. Reducing the amount of advancement of the mandible and focusing on the vertical opening may also help, but there are no studies to date to confirm this. In many cases, a simple tongue-up exercise may also be helpful. The patient is instructed to open the mouth as wide as possible. With the mouth held open, the tongue is placed up and as far back toward the soft palate as possible. While holding the tongue up in this position, the patient closes the mouth. The basis of this exercise is that it activates the muscles that retrude the mandible, thus counteracting the forces that advanced the mandible.

In some situations, patients will report that despite the feeling that the posterior teeth do not fully contact in occlusion, they would rather live with that side effect because the OA has had such a significant impact on their sleep. In these situations, the patient should be advised to continue to use the therapeutic bite rim exercise, do the tongue up exercises, and return for follow-up evaluation on a more frequent basis. It is imperative that this be documented in the patient record for medicolegal purposes. To further document the situation, photos may be taken periodically.

## Opening of interproximal contacts

There have been reports on an antidotal basis as well as clinically of a separation of contacts with the use of OAs that leads to open contacts and food catching between the teeth.

*Intervention:* The best method to prevent this side effect is to be certain that all the teeth are covered and adequately surrounded so that there is little to no chance of tooth movement. This has been reported on a very limited basis, and patients need to be advised of this potential side effect in advance as part of the informed consent form.

# CURRENT STATUS OF OAs

At this time, there are many different OA designs from which to select. The FDA currently views OAs as a singular group and does not distinguish them separately for snoring or OSA as it had done initially. In 2002, the FDA reclassified OAs as class II medical devices indicating that special controls may be needed.[26]

The FDA Web site relative to OAs has listed more than 40 OAs as being cleared and receiving a 510(k) along with the name and contact information relative to the inventor or distributor. A listing of FDA-cleared OAs can be found on the FDA Web site by inputting the user code LRK (www.accessdata.fda.gov/scripts/cdrh/cfdocs/cfPMN/pmn.cfm).

There are devices that also may be fabricated by the dentist or by a dental laboratory for individual use and are not openly advertised or marketed. In these cases, a 510(k) is not required. In many instances, an insurance company may ask for the 510(k) designation for the specific OA being utilized. Therefore, it is recommended that anyone who is providing treatment for OSA or snoring become familiar with the specific OA as it relates to the FDA.

There are numerous OAs available at this time and the majority of them are custom-fabricated. However, there are a few that are of a thermoplastic design, which are commercially available as over-the-counter (OTC) products, also termed as boil-and-bite or boil-and-fit. One study found that the OTC OAs are not as successful as the custom-fabricated OAs.[60] In addition, the OTC devices were not found to be very effective as a trial appliance, and the failure rate associated with their use was 69% as compared to a 63% success rate with custom-fabricated OAs. The lack of success was primarily related to poor retention. In addition to the findings of this study, the OTC OAs are usually designed as one-size-fits-all and consequently are usually quite bulky.

Based on the 510(k) listing by the FDA along with an awareness of the available OAs, a listing of these appliances is provided that reflects information submitted by manufacturers or inventors who responded to a request to submit information on their specific OA. The results of this inquiry are summarized here in an effort to describe many of the different devices that are available currently.

*Note:* The OAs identified in this book do not constitute a full and complete listing of all OAs currently available. The list represents those OAs from manufacturers or inventors who responded to a request for information and figures relative to their respective OA. In like manner, the listing of these OAs in no way should be construed as a recommendation for the use of any one of these OAs. The ultimate choice of an OA is the responsibility of the individual providing the service along with the comfort level and results that have been achieved with particular OAs.

## Sample of available OAs

Depending on experience and licensing, many of the OAs listed may be available from more than one dental laboratory.

Common name of OA:
    TAP© (Thornton Anterior Positioner) (Figure 11.11)
Contact information:
    866-AMISNOR
    www.amisleep.com
Type of OA design:
    Mandibular repositioning
Common name of OA:
    EMA© (Elastic Mandibular Advancement) (Figure 11.12)
Contact information:
    800–588–7898
    www.openairway.com
Type of OA design:
    Mandibular repositioning
Common name of OA:
    Klearway© (Figure 11.13)

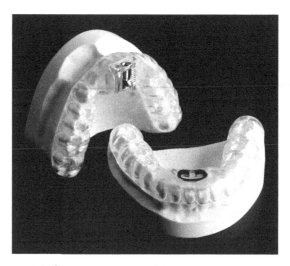

**Figure 11.11**    TAP© III Pro. (Courtesy of Airway Management Inc., 2009. Used with permission.)

Contact information:
  800–828–7626
  www.klearway.com
Type of OA design:
  Mandibular repositioning
Common name of OA:
  TheraSnore© (Figure 11.14)
Contact information:
  800–477–6673
  www.distar.com

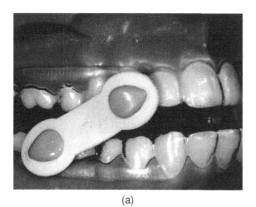

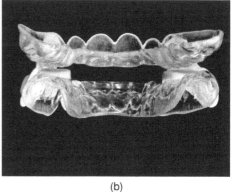

(a)                                              (b)

**Figure 11.12**    (a) Sagittal view of EMA©. (Courtesy of Frantz Design Inc., 2009. Used with permission.) (b) Lingual view of EMA©. (Courtesy of Frantz Design Inc., 2009. Used with permission.)

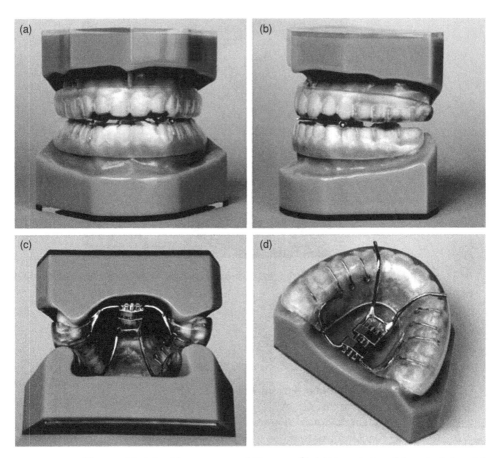

**Figure 11.13**   Various views of Klearway©. (a) Frontal view, (b) sagittal view, (c) lingual view, and (d) occlusal view of maxillary component. (Courtesy of Lowe A and Great Lakes Orthodontics Inc., 2009. Used with permission.)

Type of OA design:
    Mandibular repositioning
Common name of OA:
    PM Positioner© (Fixed and Adjustable) (Figure 11.15)
Contact information:
    800–253–1196
    www.pmpositioner.com/tech1.html
Type of OA design:
    Mandibular repositioning
Common name of OA:
    OASYS© (Oral/Nasal Airway System) (Figure 11.16)
Contact information:

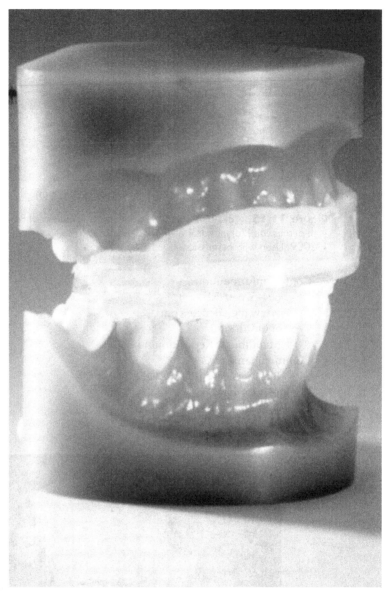

**Figure 11.14**    TheraSnore©. (Courtesy of Distar, 2009. Used with permission.)

888–866–2727
www.oasyssleep.com
Type of OA design:
    Mandibular Repositioning
Common name of OA:
    Silencer© (Figure 11.17)

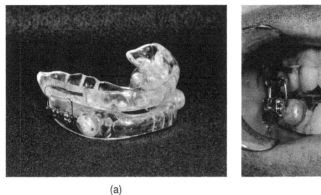
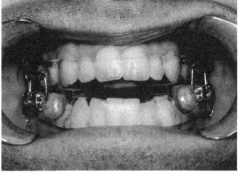

(a)                                                    (b)

**Figure 11.15**    (a) Adjustable PM Positioner©. (Courtesy of Parker J, 2009. Used with permission.) (b) Intraoral view of adjustable PM Positioner©. (Courtesy of Parker J, 2009. Used with permission.)

Contact information:
    604–576–0952
    www.the-silencer.com
Type of OA design:
    Mandibular Repositioning
Common name of OA:
    Elastomeric© (Figure 11.18)
Contact information:
    800–828–7626
    www.greatlakesortho.com

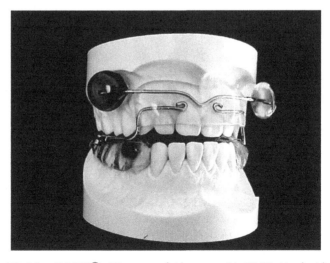

**Figure 11.16**    OASYS©. (Courtesy of Abramson M, 2009. Used with permission.)

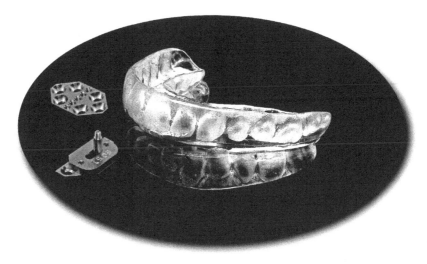

**Figure 11.17**    Silencer©. (Courtesy of Halstrom D, 2009. Used with permission.)

Type of OA design:
    Mandibular repositioning
Common name of OA:
    Herbst© (Figure 11.19)
Contact information:
    800–786–8848

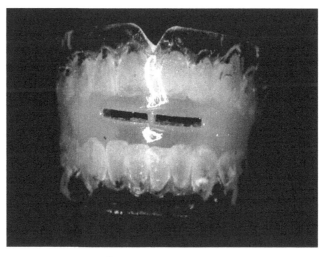

**Figure 11.18**    Elastomeric©. (Courtesy of Great Lakes Orthodontics, 2009. Used with permission.)

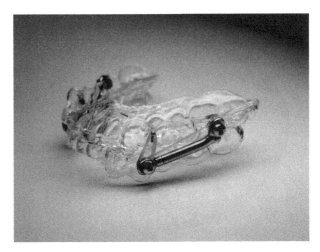

**Figure 11.19**    Thermoformed Herbst©. (Courtesy of Aleksy Kozlov, 2009. Used with permission.)

      Brabant Dental Laboratory
      Aleksey Kozlov (R&D Tech Supervisor)
Type of OA design:
      Mandibular repositioning
Common name of OA:
      Tongue Stabilizer Device (TSD) (Figures 11.20a and (11.20b)
Contact information:
      800–828–7626
      www.aveotsd.co.nz
Type of OA design:
      Tongue retainer
Common name of OA:
      SUAD© Figure (11.21)
Contact information:
      888–447–6673
      www.strongdental.com
Type of OA design:
      Mandibular repositioning
Common name of OA:
      Oral Positive Airway Pressure (OPAP) (Figure 11.22)
Contact information:
      800–786–8848
      Brabant Dental Laboratory
      Aleksey Kozlov (R&D Tech Supervisor)
Type of OA design:
      Positive airway pressure oral appliance
Common name of OA:
      TAP© with PAP (Thornton Anterior Positioner) (Figure 11.23)

(a)

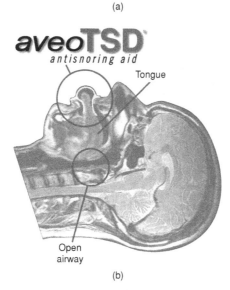

Tongue

Open
airway

(b)

**Figure 11.20** (a) aveoTSD©. (Courtesy of Innovative Health Technologies, 2009. Used with permission.) (b) aveoTSD© holding the tongue in advanced position. (Courtesy of Innovative Health Technologies, 2009. Used with permission.)

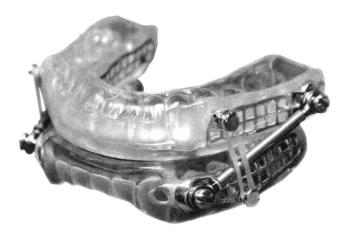

**Figure 11.21** SUAD©. (Courtesy of Strong Dental Inc., 2009. Used with permission.)

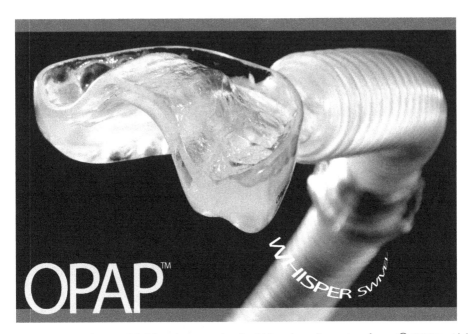

**Figure 11.22**    An example of a PAP oral appliance interface. (© OPAP—Aleksey Kozlov, 2009. Used with permission.)

Contact information:
    866-AMISNOR
    www.amisleep.com
Type of OA design:
    Mandibular repositioning combined with PAP

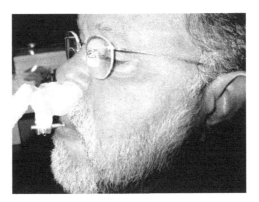

**Figure 11.23**    Combination of a TAP© oral appliance and PAP nasal pillows. (Courtesy of Airway Management Inc., 2009. Used with permission.)

## CONCLUSION

The use of OA therapy for the management of OSA and snoring is recognized as an acceptable and oftentimes appropriate treatment option. The use of these devices by a dentist who is trained in sleep medicine provides an alternative for patients who desire an alternative to PAP therapy or surgery.

The dentist who has the desire to offer this service in his or her practice will experience a great deal of satisfaction when patients report that they are sleeping better and feel more alert and energetic.

The dentist who wishes to provide this treatment needs to embark on an educational mission similar to learning about any other specialty service in dentistry. The exciting aspect to this field is the impact that results from an overall health perspective may have when an OA has contributed to the improvement in a patient's sleep, overall health, and the quality of their life.

## REFERENCES

1. Robin P. Glossoptosis due to atresia and hypotrophy of the mandible. Am J Dis Child. 1934; 48:541–547.
2. Cartwright RD and Samelson CF. The effects of a nonsurgical treatment for obstructive sleep apnea—the tongue-retaining device. JAMA. 1982; 248(6):705–709.
3. Meier-Ewert K, Schafer H, and Kloss W. Treatment of sleep apnea by a mandibular protracting device. Berichtsb 7th Eur Congr Sleep Res, Munich, Germany, 1984; 217.
4. Soll B and George P. Treatment of obstructive sleep apnea with a nocturnal airway patency appliance. N Engl J Med. 1985; 313:386–387.
5. American Sleep Disorders Association, Standards of Practice Committee. Practice parameters for the treatment of snoring and obstructive sleep apnea with oral appliances. Sleep. 1995; 18:511–513.
6. Ferguson KA, Cartwright R, Rogers R, et al. Oral appliances for snoring and obstructive sleep apnea: a review. Sleep. 2006; 29(2):244–262.
7. Kushida CA, Morgenthaler TI, Littner MR, et al. Practice parameters for the treatment of snoring and obstructive sleep apnea with oral appliances: an update for 2005. Sleep. 2006; 29(2):240–243.
8. Center for Devices and Radiologic Health, U.S. Food and Drug Administration. Class II special controls guidance document: intraoral devices for snoring and/or obstructive sleep apnea; guidance for industry and FDA. Document issued on November 12, 2002.
9. Robin P. Demonstration pratique sur la construction et la mise enbouche d'um Nouvelle appariel de redressement. Revue de Stomatologie (Paris). 1902; 9:561–590.

10. McNamara JA, ed. Naso-Respiratory Function and Craniofacial Growth. Monograph Number 9. Ann Arbor, MI: Michigan University Press. 1979; 27–40.

11. Cartwright, RD. Predicting response to the tongue retaining device for sleep apnea syndrome. Arch Otolaryngol. 1985; 111:385–388.

12. Cartwright RD, Stefoski D, Caldarelli D, et al. Toward a treatment logic for sleep apnea: the place of the tongue retaining device. Behav Res Ther. 1988; 26:121–126.

13. American Academy of Dental Sleep Medicine. AADSM treatment protocol: oral appliance therapy for sleep disordered breathing. Available at www.aadsm.org. Accessed July 12, 2009.

14. Travel TJ and Simons D. Myofascial Pain and Dysfunction: The Trigger Point Manual. Baltimore: Williams & Wilkins. 1983; 183–281, 305–320.

15. Ohayon M, Li K, and Guilleminault C. Risk factors for sleep bruxism in the general population. Chest. 2001; 119:53–61.

16. Sjoholm TT, Lowe AA, Miyamoto K, et al. Sleep bruxism in patients with sleep-disordered breathing. Arch Oral Biol. 2000; 45:889–896.

17. White D. Pharyngeal resistance in normal humans: influence of gender, age and obesity. J Appl Physiol. 1985; 58:365–371.

18. Schwab R. Imaging for the snoring and sleep apnea patient. In: Attanasio R and Bailey D, eds. Sleep Disorders: Dentistry's Role (Dental Clinics of North America; 45:4). Philadelphia: WB Saunders. 2001; 759–796.

19. Ferguson KA, Love LL, and Ryan CF. Effect of mandibular and tongue protrusion on upper airway size. Am J Respir Crit Care Med. 1997; 155:1748–1754.

20. Isono S, Tanaka A, Sho Y, et al. Advancement of the mandible improves velopharyngeal airway patency. J Appl Physiol. 1995; 79:2132–2138.

21. Ishida M, Inoue Y, Suto Y, et al. Mechanism of action and therapeutic indication of prosthetic mandibular advancement in obstructive sleep apnea syndrome. Psychiatry Clin Neurosci. 1998; 52:227–229.

22. Tsuiki S, Hiyama S, Ono T, et al. Effects of a titratable oral appliance on supine airway size in awake non-apneic individuals. Sleep. 2001; 24:554–560.

23. Tsuiki S, Lowe AA, Almeida FR, et al. Effects of an anteriorly titrated mandibular position on awake airway and obstructive sleep apnea severity. Am J Orthod Dentofacial Orthop. 2004; 125:548–555.

24. Gale DJ, Sawyer RH, Woodcock A, et al. Do oral appliances enlarge the airway in patients with obstructive sleep apnoea? A prospective computerized tomographic study. Eur J Orthod. 2000; 22:159–168.

25. Eveloff SE, Rosenberg CL, Carlisle CC, et al. Efficacy of a Herbst mandibular advancement device in obstructive sleep apnea. Am J Respir Crit Care Med. 1994; 149:905–909.

26. de Almedia FR, Bittencourt LR, de Almeida CIR, et al. Effects of mandibular posture on obstructive sleep apnea severity and the temporomandibular joint in patients fitted with an oral appliance. Sleep. 2002; 25(5):507–513.

27. Walker-Engstrom ML, Ringqvist I, Vestling O, et al. A prospective randomized study comparing two different degrees of mandibular advancement with a dental appliance in treatment of severe obstructive sleep apnea. Sleep Breath. 2003; 7:119–130.

28. Rose E, Staats R, Virchow C, et al. A comparative study of two mandibular advancement appliances for the treatment of obstructive sleep apnea. Eur J Orthod. 2002; 24:191–198.

29. Marklund M, Sahlin C, Stenlund H, et al. Mandibular advancement device in patients with obstructive sleep apnea: long-term effects on apnea and sleep. Chest. 2001; 120:162–169.

30. George P. Selecting sleep-disordered-breathing appliances: biomechanical considerations. JADA. 2001; 132:339–347.

31. Ono T, Lowe AA, Ferguson KA, et al. A tongue retaining device and sleep-state genioglossus muscle activity in patients with obstructive sleep apnea. Angle Orthod. 1996; 66:273–280.

32. Yoshida K. Effect of a prosthetic appliance for treatment of sleep apnea syndrome on masticatory and tongue muscle activity. J Prosth Dent. 1998; 79:537–544.

33. Tsuiki S, de Almeida FR, Bhalla F, et al. Supine dependent changes in upper airway size in awake obstructive sleep apnea patients. Sleep Breath. 2003; 7:43–50.

34. Hoffstein V. Review of oral appliances for treatment of sleep-disordered breathing. Sleep Breath. 2007; 11:1–22.

35. Barnes M, McEvoy RD, Banks S, et al. Efficacy of positive airway pressure and oral appliance in mild to moderate obstructive sleep apnea. Am J Respir Crit Care Med. 2004; 170:656–664.

36. Gotsopoulos H, Chen C, Qian J, et al. Oral appliance therapy improves symptoms in obstructive sleep apnea: a randomized, controlled trial. Am J Respir Crit Care Med. 2002; 166:743–748.

37. Tan YK, L'Estrange RP, Luo YM, et al. Mandibular advancement splints and continuous positive airway pressure in patients with obstructive sleep apnoea: a randomized cross-over trial. Eur J Orthod. 2002; 24:239–249.

38. Gotsopoulos H, Kelly JJ, and Cistulli PA. Oral appliance therapy reduces blood pressure in obstructive sleep apnea: a randomized, controlled trial. Sleep. 2004; 27:934–941.

39. Yoshida K. Effect on blood pressure of oral appliance therapy for sleep apnea syndrome. Int J Prosthodont. 2006; 19:61–66.

40. Itzhaki S, Dorchin H, Clark G, et al. The effects of 1-year treatment with a Herbst mandibular advancement splint on obstructive sleep apnea, oxidative stress, and endothelial function. Chest. 2007; 131:740–749.

41. Ferguson K, Ono T, Lowe A, et al. A randomized crossover study of an oral appliance vs nasal continuous positive airway pressure in the treatment of mild-moderate obstructive sleep apnea. Chest. 1996; 109:1269–1275.

42. Ferguson KA, Ono T, Lowe AA, et al. A short term controlled trial of an adjustable oral appliance for the treatment of mild to moderate obstructive sleep apnoea. Thorax. 1997; 52:362–368.

43. Engleman HM, McDonald JP, Graham D, et al. Randomized crossover trial of two treatments for sleep apnea/hypopnea syndrome: continuous positive airway pressure and mandibular repositioning splint. Am J Respir Crit Care Med. 2002; 166:855–859.

44. Randerath WJ, Heise M, Hinz R, et al. An individually adjustable oral appliance vs continuous positive airway pressure in mild-to-moderate obstructive sleep apnea syndrome. Chest. 2002; 122:569–575.

45. Clark GT, Blumenthal I, Yoffe N, et al. A crossover study comparing the efficacy of continuous positive airway pressure with anterior mandibular positioning devices on patients with obstructive sleep apnea. Chest. 1996; 109:1477–1483.

46. McGowen AD, Makker HK, Battagel JM, et al. Long-term use of mandibular advancement splints for snoring and obstructive sleep apnea: a questionnaire survey. Eur Respir J. 2001; 17:462–466.

47. Wilhelmsson B, Tegelberg A, Walker-Engstrom ML, et al. A prospective randomized study of a dental appliance compared with uvulopalatopharyngoplasty in the treatment of obstructive sleep apnoea. Acta Otolaryngol. 1999; 119:503–509.

48. Tegelberg A, Wilhelmsson B, Walker-Engstrom ML, et al. Effects and adverse events of a dental appliance for treatment of obstructive sleep apnoea. Swed Dent J. 1999; 23:117–126.

49. Walker-Engstrom ML, Wilhelmsson B, Tegelberg A, et al. Quality of life assessment of treatment with dental appliance or UPPP in patients with mild to moderate obstructive sleep apnoea: a prospective randomized 1-year follow-up study. J Sleep Res. 2000; 9:303–308.

50. Ringqvist M, Walker-Engstrom ML, Tegelberg A, et al. Dental and skeletal changes after 4 years of obstructive sleep apnea treatment with a mandibular advancement device: a prospective, randomized study. Am J Orthod Dentofacial Orthop. 2003; 124:53–60.

51. Walker-Engstrom ML, Tegelberg A, Wilhelmsson B, et al. 4-year follow-up of treatment with dental appliance or uvulopalatopharyngoplasty in patients with obstructive sleep apnea: a randomized study. Chest. 2002; 121:739–746.

52. Hoekema A, de Lange J, Stegenga B, et al. Oral appliances and maxillomandibular advancement surgery: an alternative treatment protocol for an obstructive sleep apnea-hypopnea syndrome. J Oral Maxillofac Surg. 2006; 64:886–891.

53. Mehta A, Qian J, Petocz P, et al. A randomized, controlled study of a mandibular advancement splint for obstructive sleep apnea. Am J Respir Crit Care Med. 2001; 163:1457–1461.

54. Esaki K, Kanegae H, Uchida T, et al. Treatment of sleep apnea with a new separated type of dental appliance (mandibular advancing positioned). Kurume Med J. 1997; 44:315–319.

55. Marklund M, Franklin KA, Sahlin C, et al. The effect of a mandibular advancement device on apneas and sleep in patients with obstructive sleep apnea. Chest. 1998; 113:707–713.

56. Frantz D. The difference between success and failure. Sleep Rev. 2001; 2:20–23.

57. Pitsis AJ, Darendeliler MA, Gotsopoulos H, et al. Effect of vertical dimension on efficacy of oral appliance therapy in obstructive sleep apnea. Am J Respir Crit Care Med. 2002; 166:860–864.

58. Collup NA, Anderson WM, Boehlecke B, et al. Clinical guidelines for the use of unattended portable monitors in the diagnosis of obstructive sleep apnea in adult patients. J Clin Sleep Med. 2007; 3(7):737–747.

59. de Almeida FR, Lowe AA, Tsuiki S, et al. Long-term compliance and side effects of oral appliances used for the treatment of snoring and obstructive sleep apnea syndrome. J Clin Sleep Med. 2005; 1:143–152.

60. Vanderveken OM, Devolder A, Marklund M, et al. Comparison of a custom-made and a thermoplastic oral appliance for the treatment of mild sleep apnea. Am J Respir Crit Care Med. 2008; 178:197–202.

# Appendices

# Appendix 1: Abbreviations for sleep medicine

The following is a listing of abbreviations that are used in sleep medicine and may be commonly encountered by the dentist:

| | |
|---|---|
| AASM | American Academy of Sleep Medicine |
| ADD | attention-deficit disorder |
| ADHD | attention-deficit hyperactivity disorder |
| AHI | apnea–hypopnea index |
| APAP | autoadjusting positive airway pressure |
| BiPAP | bilevel positive airway pressure |
| BMI | body mass index |
| CHF | congestive heart failure |
| CPAP | continuous positive airway pressure |
| CRSD | circadian rhythm sleep disorders |
| CSA | central sleep apnea |
| DA | dopamine |
| *DSM* | *Diagnostic and Statistical Manual of Mental Disorders* |
| DSPD | delayed sleep phase disorder |
| ECG | electrocardiogram |
| EDS | excessive daytime sleepiness |
| EEG | electroencephalogram/electroencephalography |
| EMG | electromyogram |
| EOG | electrooculogram |
| ESS | Epworth Sleepiness Scale |
| FDA | Federal Drug Administration |
| GABA | $\gamma$-aminobutyric acid |
| GERD | gastroesophageal reflux disease |
| *ICSD* | *International Classification of Sleep Disorders* |
| *ICSD-2* | *International Classification of Sleep Disorders, Second Edition* |

| | |
|---|---|
| MRA | mandibular repositioning appliance |
| MRI | magnetic resonance imaging |
| MSLT | Multiple Sleep Latency Test |
| MWT | Maintenance of Wakefulness Test |
| NE | norepinephrine |
| NREM | nonrapid eye movement |
| NSF | National Sleep Foundation |
| OA | oral appliance |
| OSA | obstructive sleep apnea |
| PAP | positive airway pressure |
| PLMD | periodic limb movement disorder |
| PLMS | periodic limb movements during sleep (or PLM) |
| PSG | polysomnogram/polysomnography (sleep study) |
| REM | rapid eye movement |
| RERA | respiratory effort-related arousal |
| RLS | restless legs syndrome |
| RMMA | rhythmic masticatory muscle activity |
| SRBD | sleep-related breathing disorders |
| SRED | sleep-related eating disorder |
| SSRI | selective serotonin reuptake inhibitor |
| SSS | Stanford Sleepiness Scale |
| TMD | temporomandibular disorders |
| TMJ | temporomandibular joint |
| TRD | tongue-retaining device |
| UARS | upper airway resistance syndrome |
| UPPP | uvulopalatopharyngoplasty |

# Appendix 2: Glossary of terms for sleep medicine

The following is a listing of terms that are used in sleep medicine and may be commonly encountered by the dentist:

**Advanced sleep phase syndrome:** The sleep–wake times are earlier than the accepted times, which results in earlier bedtimes and earlier awakenings.

**Apnea:** Historically defined as the total cessation of breathing for 10 seconds or longer. In sleep medicine, apnea is a reduction or cessation of 70% or greater in airflow for 10 seconds or more.

**Apnea–hypopnea index (AHI):** The average number of apneas and hypopneas per hour of sleep.

**Arousal:** An abrupt or sudden change from a deep stage of sleep to a lighter stage of sleep, or from REM sleep to wakefulness.

**Cataplexy:** A finding oftentimes found in narcolepsy. A sudden loss of muscle tone associated with an emotional event such as laughter, surprise, excitement, or even anger.

**Circadian rhythm:** Oftentimes referred to as one's internal clock. Associated with the light–dark cycle and occurs over about a 24-hour period.

**Deep sleep/delta sleep:** Oftentimes referred to as restorative sleep. This is associated with delta waves on an EEG. In the sleep study, this is known as stage N3 (may also be termed NREM stages 3 and 4). In some situations, deep sleep is associated with REM sleep because the ability to be awakened is more difficult.

**Delayed sleep phase syndrome:** The sleep–wake times are delayed, which may make it difficult to fall asleep at the normal times, and awakenings are later.

**Drowsiness:** A state of quiet wakefulness that is seen or experienced prior to sleep onset.

**Epoch:** Refers to the amount of time that sleep is being recorded during a sleep study, typically for 20- or 30-second intervals.

**Fatigue:** The feeling of low energy levels, listlessness, or low motivation to be active with the inability to be sleepy or fall asleep.

**Fragmentation (sleep fragmentation):** The presence of an interruption of any stage of sleep by the appearance or presentation of a different sleep stage or by the onset of wakefulness.

**Hypercapnia:** An elevation of $CO_2$ levels in the blood.

**Hypersomnia—excessive sleepiness or excessive daytime sleepiness (EDS):** The feeling of sleepiness at times when an individual should not be sleepy. Can also be associated with prolonged sleep.

**Hypnagogic hallucinations:** Images that may be visual, auditory, or tactile, which occur at the onset of sleep and may be related to the onset of REM.

**Hypnopomic hallucinations:** These are events that occur at a time when there is a transition from sleep to wakefulness.

**Hypocretin (also known as Orexin):** A neurochemical associated with the control of sleep. Oftentimes associated with narcolepsy and more common when cataplexy is present.

**Hypopnea:** A reduction in airflow by 30% or greater associated with a similar reduction in thoracoabdominal movement and a 4% or greater fall in the blood oxygen level as measured by oximetry.

**Insomnia:** The inability to initiate or maintain sleep and associated with sleep loss.

**K-complex:** A distinct sharp EEG waveform associated with stage N2 (NREM stage 2) sleep.

**Light sleep:** Often associated with stage N1 (NREM stage 1) sleep and at times with stage N2 (NREM stage 2) sleep.

**Maintenance of Wakefulness Test (MWT):** A daytime test that assesses the ability of an individual to remain awake when reclined in a darkened room. This test is oftentimes used to determine the success of therapy for sleep apnea and the resolution of daytime sleepiness by the ability to remain awake. May be associated with excessive sleepiness.

**Multiple Sleep Latency Test (MSLT):** A form of daytime testing consisting of a series of 4 or 5 times (naps) that determine the propensity to fall asleep. This is used to test for the risk of narcolepsy and the onset of REM (stage R) within a 15-minute period.

**Nightmare:** An unpleasant/frightening dream that is associated with REM sleep.

**NREM (Non-REM) sleep:** Nonrapid eye movement sleep that is composed of three stages (N1, N2, and N3). These stages occur 4–6 times during a normal night's sleep.

**Parasomnia:** A disorder of sleep associated with arousal(s) or the transition between different sleep stages. Typically an event that disrupts sleep (sleepwalking, sleeptalking).

**Periodic breathing (Cheyne–Stokes respiration):** A type of breathing pattern that is a crescendo–decrescendo type of respiration.

**Periodic limb movement (PLM):** Also referred to as periodic limb movement disorder (PLMD) during a sleep study. An involuntary movement, usually of the leg, that occurs during sleep. May also involve flexion of the foot or extension of the large toe.

**Polysomnogram (PSG—also known as a sleep study):** Done during sleep (overnight) and records multiple physiologic events during sleep.

**Rapid eye movement (REM) sleep:** A period of sleep when the eyes typically move rapidly and the body is in a paralyzed state. Also known as *paradoxical sleep.*

**Respiratory disturbance index (RDI):** The apnea–hypopnea index (AHI) that also includes the RERAs.

**Respiratory effort-related arousals (RERAs):** A respiratory event that is associated with an arousal (change in sleep state) but cannot be scored on the sleep study as an apnea or hypopnea.

**Sleep efficiency:** Usually measured in percent and is the amount of recorded time asleep to the amount of time in bed. The normal is considered to be 85%.

**Sleep hygiene:** The habits and lifestyle that contribute to good sleep, such as room temperature, noise, and the amount of light.

**Sleep latency:** The time between when the lights are turned off and the presentation of sleep or a given sleep stage such as REM sleep (REM sleep latency).

**Sleep onset:** The amount of time observed on a sleep study that it typically takes to go from wakefulness to N1 (NREM stage 1) sleep.

**Sleep paralysis:** A stage observed between sleep and wakefulness associated with the inability to move (atonia) or speak. Considered to be associated with REM sleep and can be frightening, especially if breathing is also affected.

**Sleep–wake cycle:** The internal clock control of the sleep and wakefulness cycle (circadian rhythm).

**Slow-wave sleep:** Also referred to as delta sleep, stage N3 (NREM stages 3 and 4), or restorative sleep. This is associated with slower EEG waves as seen on the sleep study.

**Snoring:** The noise associated with respiration during inspiration that is caused by vibration of the unsupported soft tissues in the upper airway (soft palate, uvula, and oropharyngeal tissues). This is often associated with an incomplete obstruction but may also be a symptom of sleep apnea.

**Total sleep time (TST):** The total amount of time actually spent in the sleep state (total of REM and NREM sleep).

**Upper airway resistance syndrome (UARS):** Events that do not seemingly meet the criteria for apnea and hypopnea but appear as RERAs on a sleep study. It appears similar to sleep apnea, but oftentimes the blood oxygen level does not drop.

**Zeitgeber:** (German for "time givers") A cue found in the environment (sunlight, social interaction, noise, or an alarm clock) that allows an individual to entrain to their circadian (24-hour clock) rhythm.

# Index

Printed in the United States
By Bookmasters